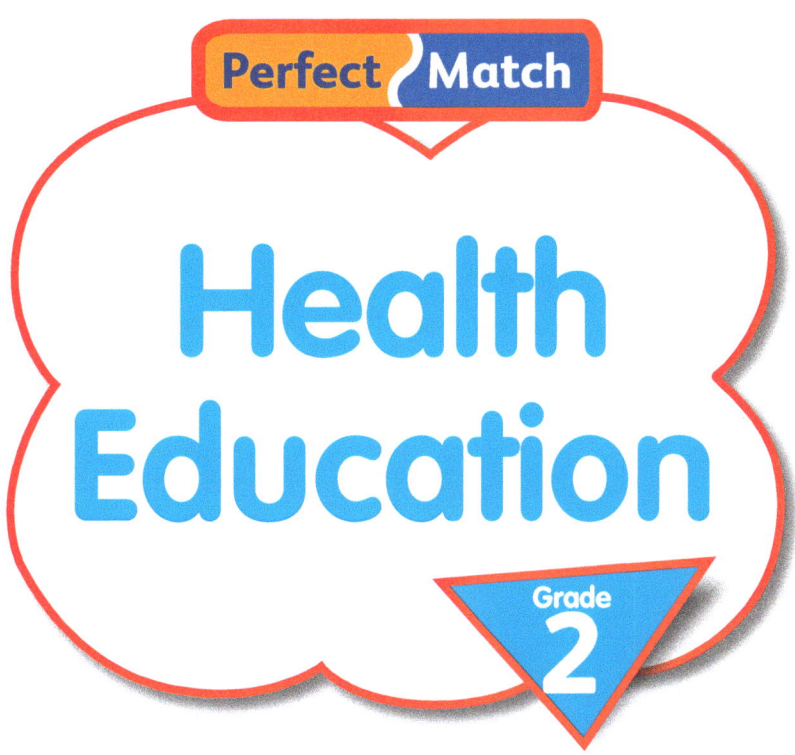

Dr Michael Chia

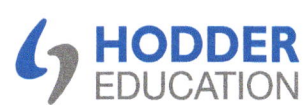

Hachette UK's policy is to use papers that are natural, renewable and recyclable products and made from wood grown in well-managed forests and other controlled sources. The logging and manufacturing processes are expected to conform to the environmental regulations of the country of origin.

ISBN: 978 981 47 6773 6

© Dr Michael Chia 2007, 2018

First published in 2007 by Pearson Education South Asia Pte Ltd

This new edition published in 2018 by
Hachette Singapore Private Limited
Published from 2023 by Hodder Education,
An Hachette UK Company
Carmelite House
50 Victoria Embankment
London EC4Y 0DZ
www.hoddereducation.com

Impression number   10 9 8 7 6 5
Year   2023

All rights reserved. Apart from any use permitted under UK copyright law, no part of this publication may be reproduced or transmitted in any form or by any means, electronic or mechanical, including photocopying and recording, or held within any information storage and retrieval system, without permission in writing from the publisher or under licence from the Copyright Licensing Agency Limited. Further details of such licences (for reprographic reproduction) may be obtained from the Copyright Licensing Agency Limited, www.cla.co.uk

Printed in Singapore

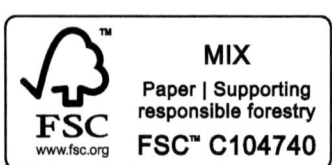

Contents

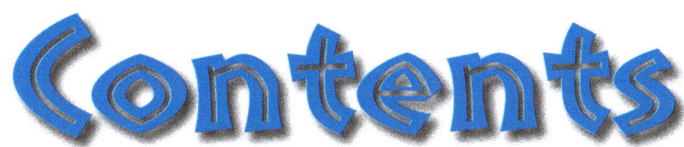
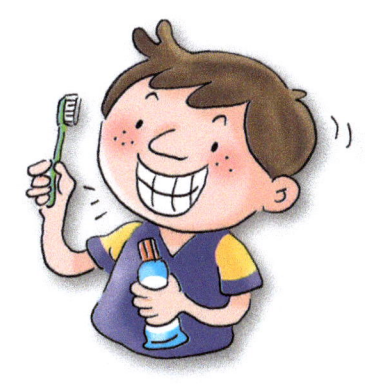

Physical Health

Lesson	Title	Page
1	Growing Well	3
2	More About Food	5
3	Find Your Balance	7
4	Snack Attack!	9
5	Fruit And Vegetables	11
6	Healthy Food Choices	13
7	Eyes, Ears And Nose	15
8	Sleep Well And Learn Better	17
9	Stop Spreading Germs	19
10	Gums, Teeth And Tongue	21
11	Brush Your Teeth And Gums	25

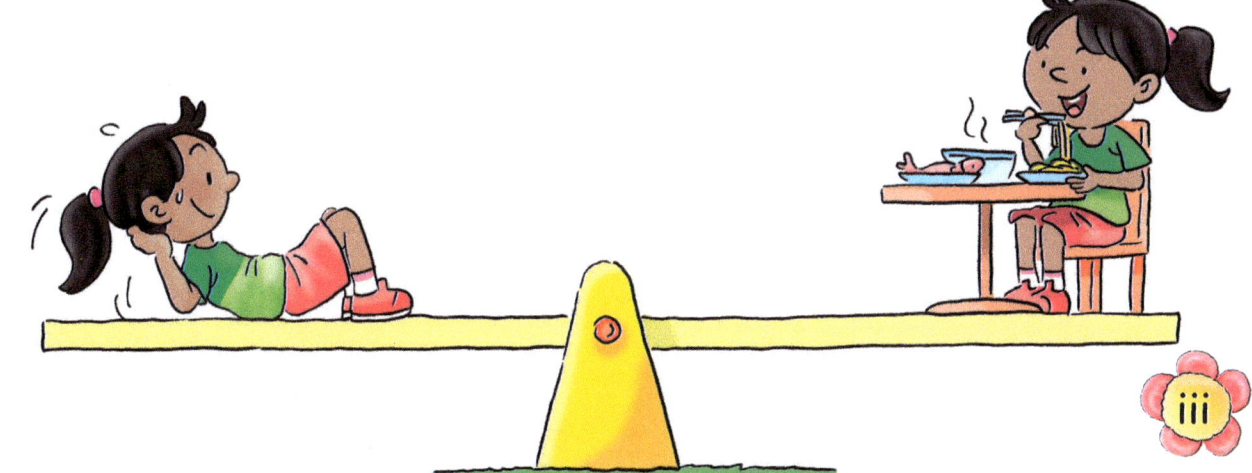

Environment And Your Health

Lesson	Title	Page
1	Crossing Safely	29
2	What Went Wrong?	31
3	Safety Rules I	33
4	Safety Rules II	35
5 & 6	Road Safety First	37
7	Germs Can Make You Sick	39
8	Germs Are Everywhere	41
9	Do Not Share Your Germs	43

Emotional And Psychological Health

Lesson	Title	Page
1	Not Happy At All	47
2	Dealing With Anger	49
3	Lam's Story	51
4	Caring For Others	53
5	Crack The Code!	55
6	Wonderful Words	57
7	Leave Me Alone!	59
8	Bullying And Teasing	61
9	How To Tackle Bullying	63

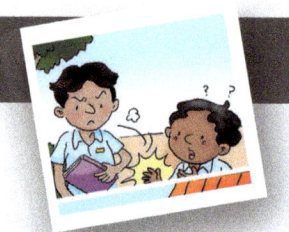

Learning Log — 65-70

Introduction to the Pupil's Book

The **Perfect Match** Primary Health Education Pupil's Book is a full-colour textbook-cum-activity book. It contains lessons based on topics from the three dimensions in Health Education: Physical Health, Environment and Your Health, and Emotional and Psychological Health.

The book is organised by dimension and is presented in the order stated above. The pages in each dimension are colour-coded for easy reference.

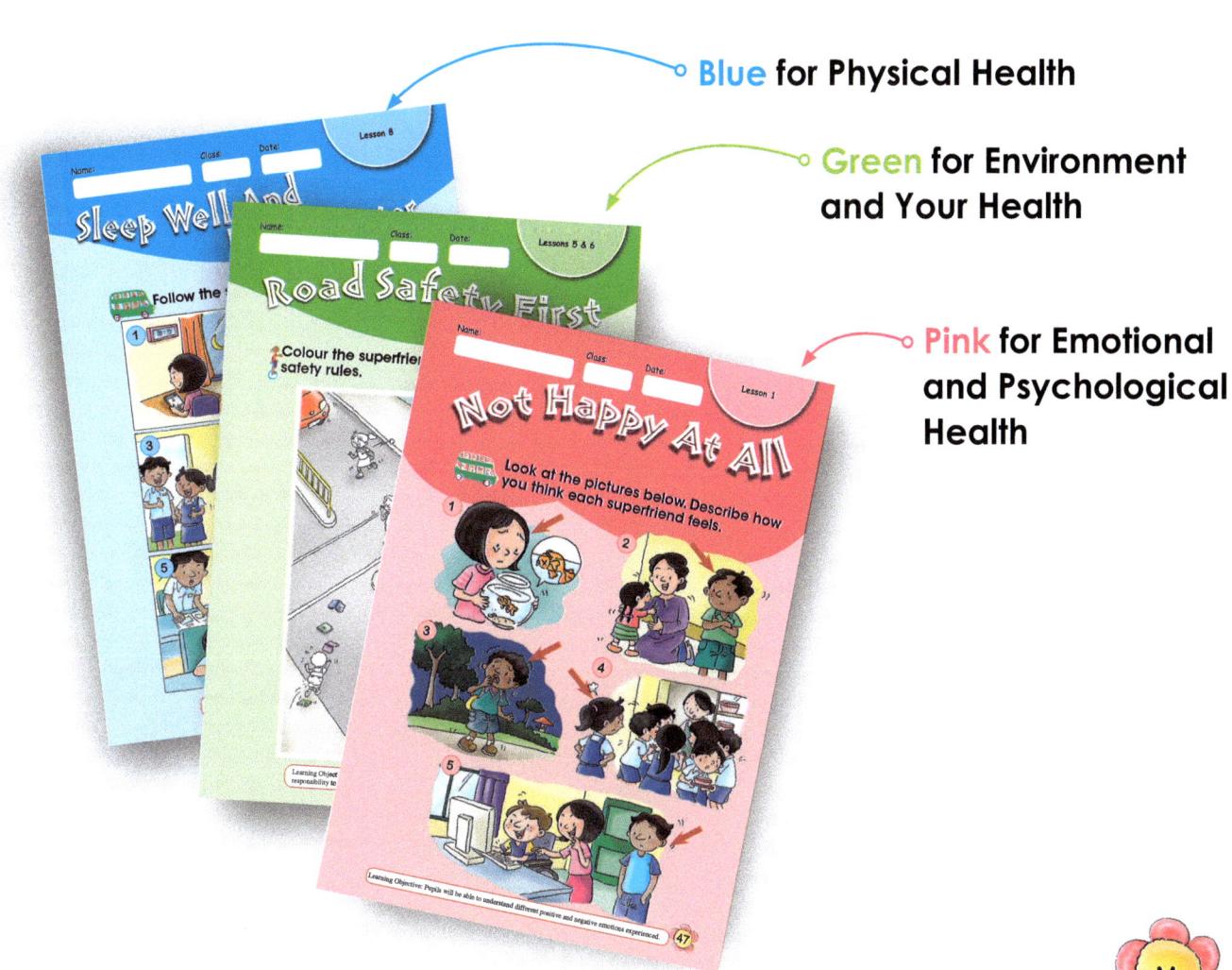

Blue for Physical Health

Green for Environment and Your Health

Pink for Emotional and Psychological Health

The Pupil's Book contains a variety of activities such as role plays, surveys, songs, matching exercises and craft work. In addition, there is a mix of activities requiring work in pairs, in groups or with the class.

Four icons indicate the nature of the activity to be conducted.

individual work

pair work

group work

class work

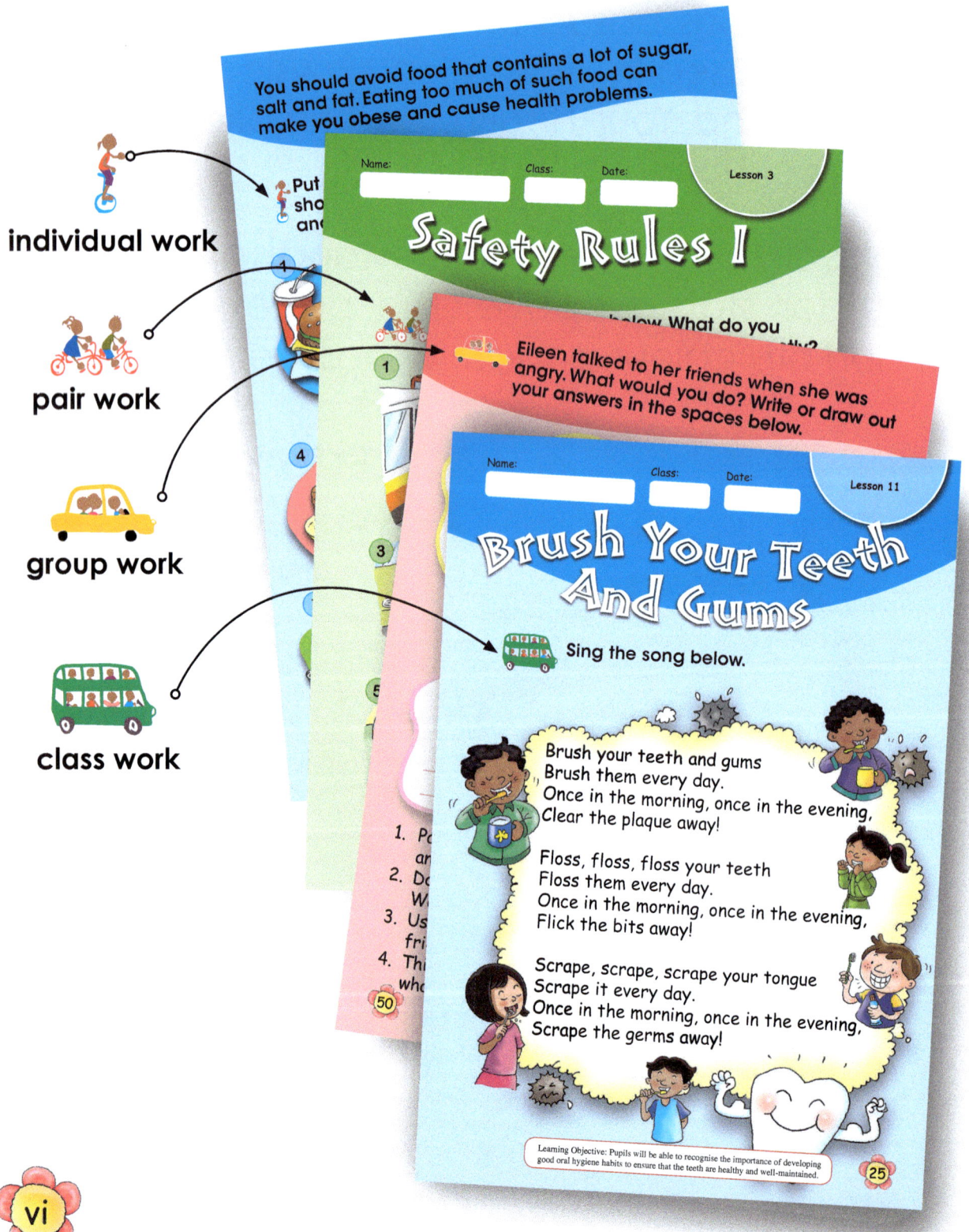

Difficult terms mentioned in the text are explained through a feature signalled by the dictionary icon.

The learning objective(s) for each lesson is/are listed for parents' and teachers' reference.

A dictionary icon signals the explanation of any difficult term(s) found on the page.

The learning objective(s) for each lesson is/are indicated at the opening page of each lesson.

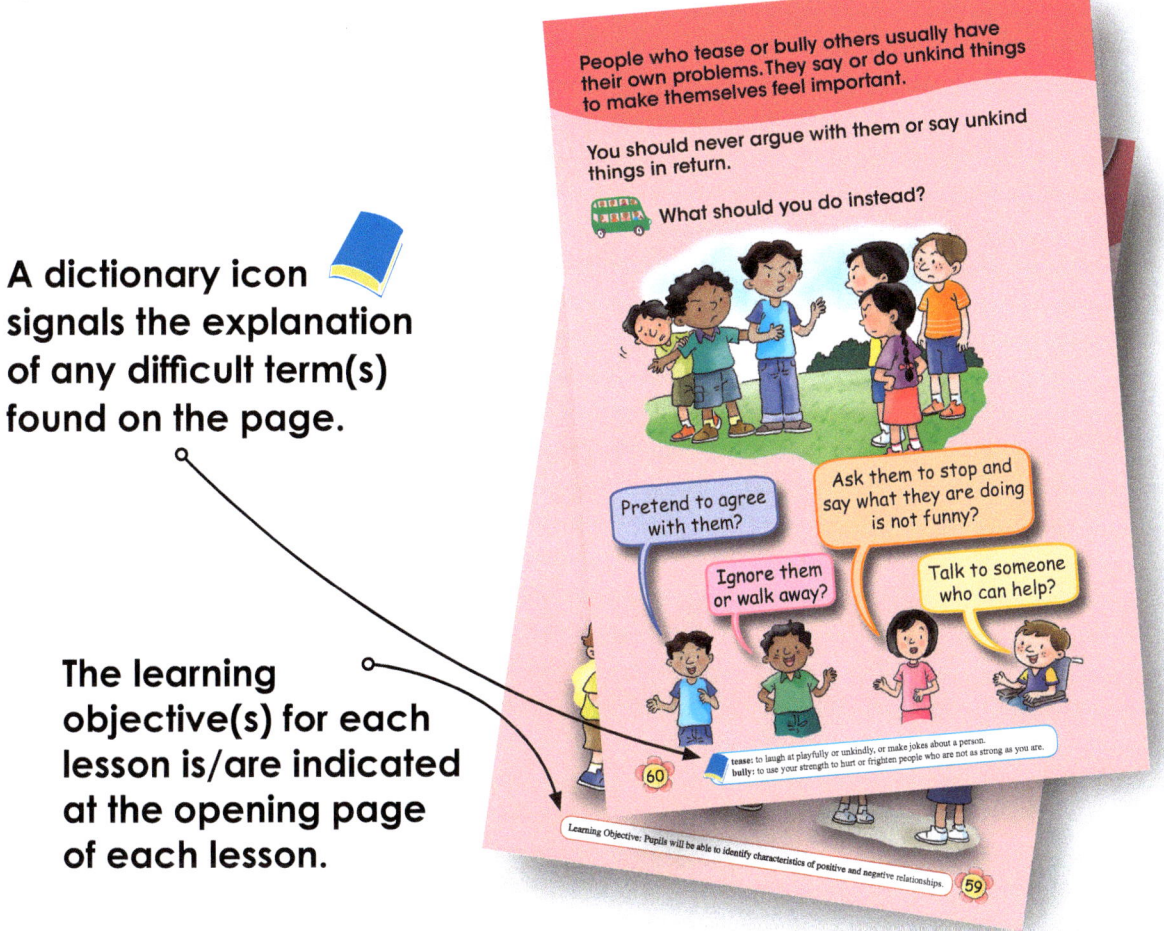

A Note on Short Forms: In the first three books, short-forms of verbs are avoided as early users of the language may not have knowledge of them. In Books 4, 5 and 6, these contractions are present throughout so that the language flows more naturally and pupils can become more acquainted with real English use.

A Learning Log has been added at the end of the book to give opportunity for reflective learning.

Introduction to the Superfriends

The materials in the Perfect Match **Perfect Match** Primary Health Education Pupil's Book revolve around six superfriends from some of the ASEAN countries. These six friends will accompany the pupils in the learning process as they move from Book 1 to 6. The first letters of their names — Haris, Eileen, Ajit, Lam, Tawan and Harold — form the word 'h-e-a-l-t-h'.

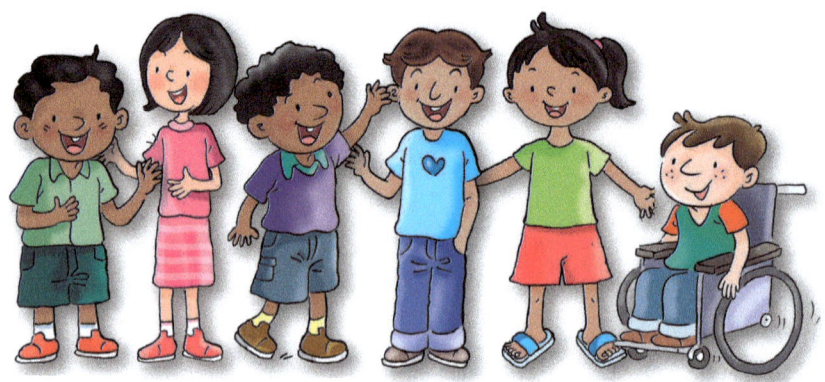

Taking the cue from the World Health Organization (WHO) to build 'a better and healthier future for people all over the world', the superfriends come together from different ASEAN countries to help young people like themselves develop healthy habits to ensure a better future. This health series aims to help pupils start early in health education, to keep themselves well physically, psychologically and emotionally. In addition, they will also learn to behave responsibly in order to enhance the environment in their home countries.

Hi, I am Haris.

Haris is a well-built Malaysian boy. He is the wise one among the superfriends. He is fun and peace-loving and tries his best to keep the people around him happy.

"Hi, I am Eileen."

Eileen is a tall slim Singaporean girl. She loves Maths and Science and knows a lot about computers. Eileen enjoys helping her friends with school work.

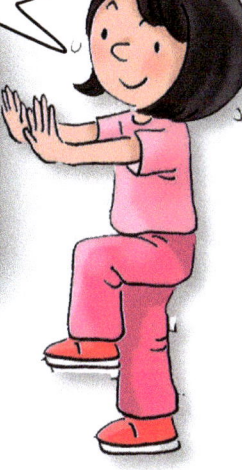

"Hi, I am Ajit."

Ajit is a Malaysian boy who loves reading and has a flair for languages. He speaks well and is always eager to listen to his friends when they have problems.

"Hi, I am Lam."

Lam is a Vietnamese boy who is active and full of ideas. He loves school and hopes to be a teacher when he grows up. He is good-natured and patient and is extremely well-liked.

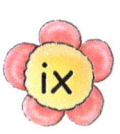

Hi, I am Tawan.

Tawan is an athletic and sporty Thai girl who also loves art. She is the most physically active and well-rounded person in the group. She is smart and strong in character but also fun-loving and witty.

Hi, I am Harold.

Harold has a Canadian father and a biracial mother who is half Singaporean. He is musically talented and has great willpower. Despite his disability, he has never felt disadvantaged and he always encourages his friends to pursue their interests.

About The Author

Dr Michael Chia is Professor of Paediatric Exercise Science at the Physical Education & Sports Science Group in the National Institute of Education (NIE), Nanyang Technological University (NTU). He is an established author in the field of Health Education, Physical Education and Sports Science.

His health education publications include *Healthy, Well and Wise: Take PRIDE For A Life of Wellness, Invest in Better Health* and *Treks: All Aboard!*.

Physical Health

In this section, you will learn about:

- good eating habits;
- the importance of physical activities and sleep;
- taking good care of your eyes, ears and nose;
- germs and how they spread disease; and
- caring for your mouth.

Name: Class: Date: **Lesson 1**

Growing Well

Listen carefully to your teacher. Circle 'B' if Ajit and Tawan had breakfast, 'L' if they had lunch, 'D' if they had dinner, and 'E' if they exercised.

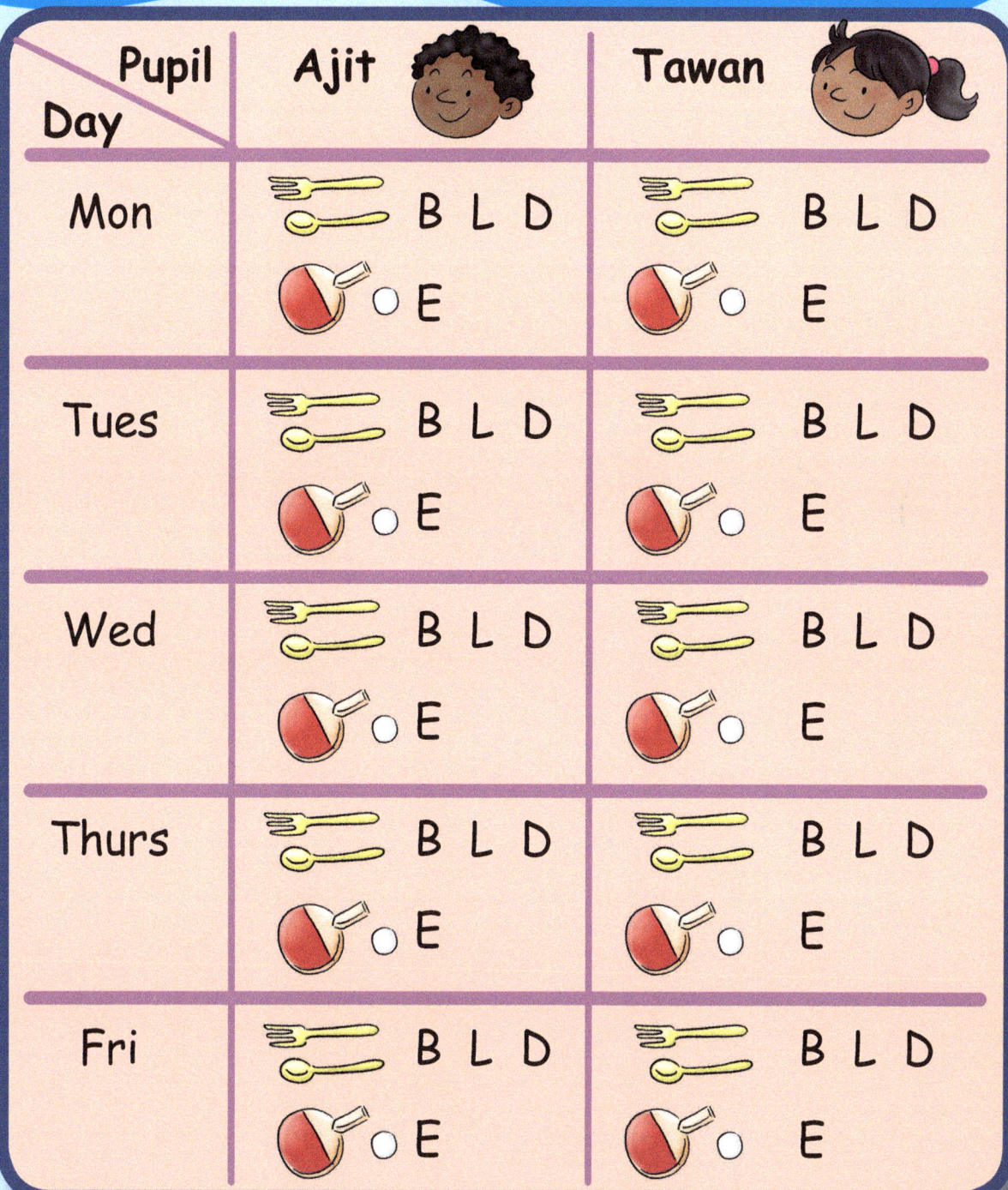

Learning Objective: Pupils will be able to understand how to achieve healthy growth.

To grow well, you need regular meals and exercise.

Record your meals and exercise for the next five days. Circle the letters 'B', 'L', 'D', and 'E'.

B: breakfast   L: lunch   D: dinner   E: exercise

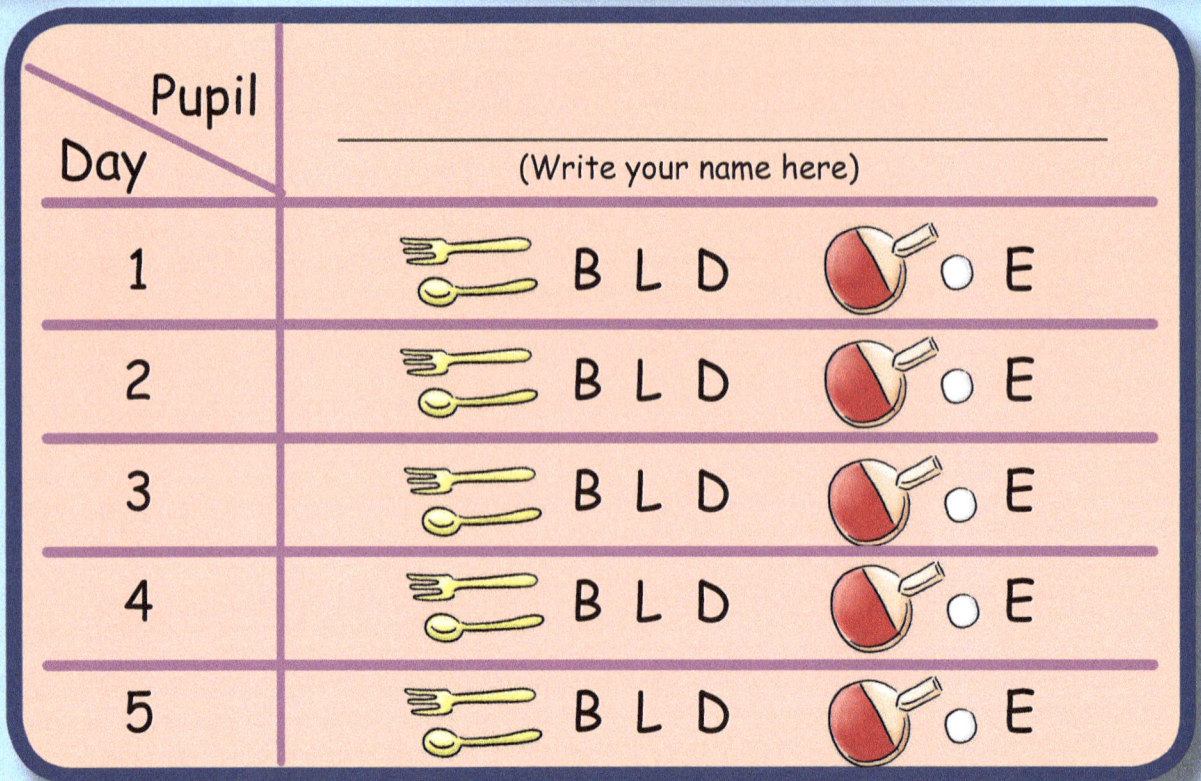

1. Which meals did you have every day?

_____

2. How many times did you exercise in the five days?

_____

Name: Class: Date: Lesson 2

More About Food

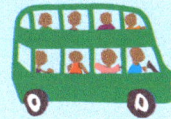 Eileen, Haris and Ajit are at a food centre. Read what they are saying.

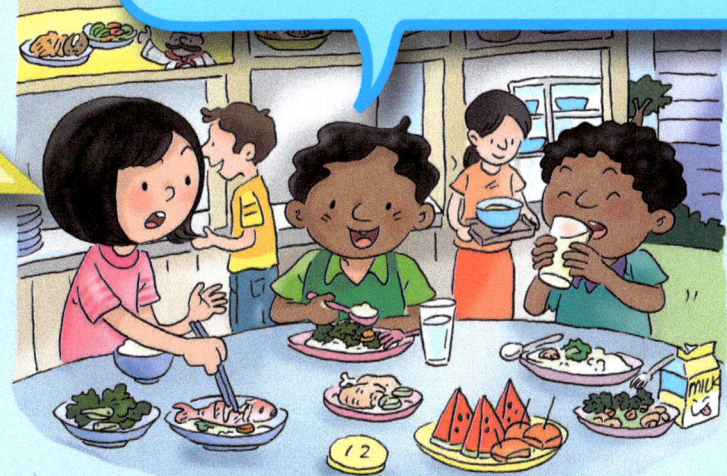

"My favourite is rice and vegetables. I have vegetables at every meal."

"Look at all the different food we are having."

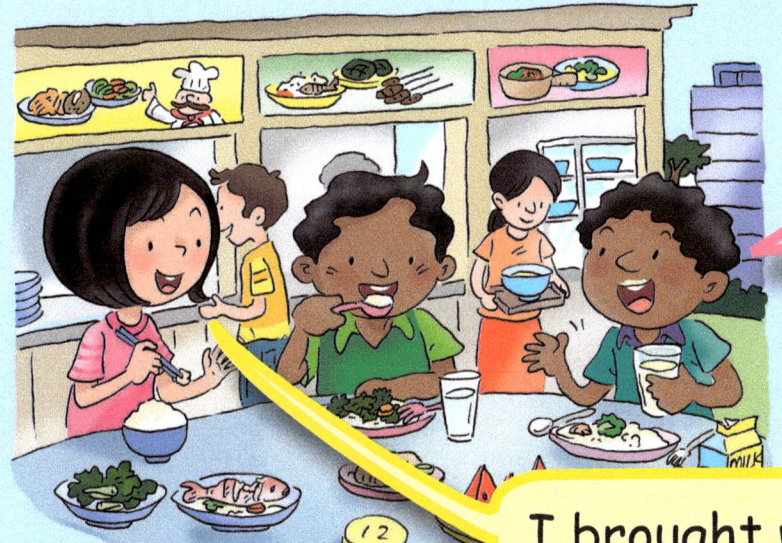

"Me too! I also need a glass of milk at every meal. Hey Eileen, you do not have a drink!"

"I brought water from home. I will have some later."

Learning Objective: Pupils will be able to understand how to achieve healthy growth.

Did you see how many types of food Eileen, Haris and Ajit were having? You must eat different types of food to stay healthy.

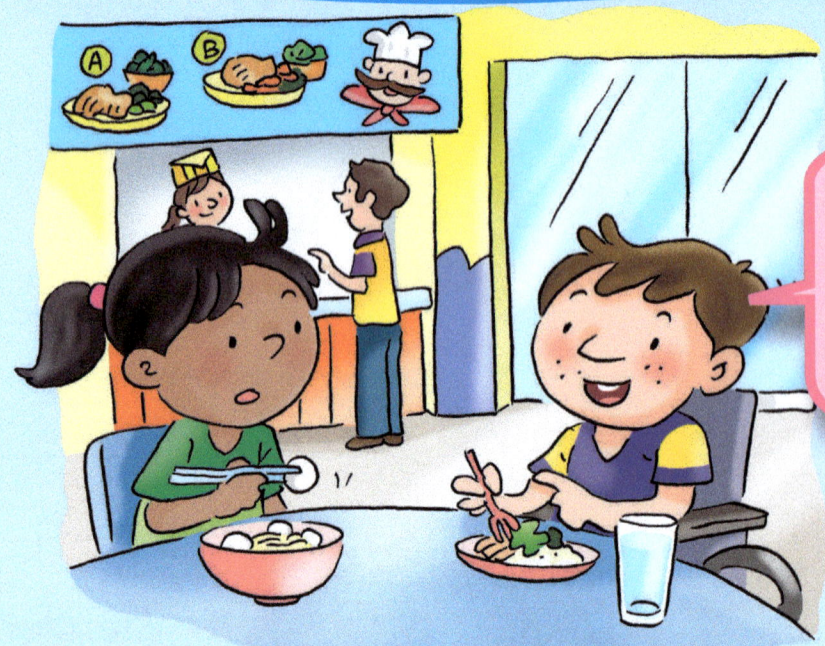

I know you love fishball noodles, but do not eat them every day.

Drink at least eight glasses of water every day. If the weather is hot or you are exercising, drink more. The colour of your urine must be a very light yellow because that shows you have enough water to function well.

Draw and describe the types of food you eat. They can be from the school canteen or from home.

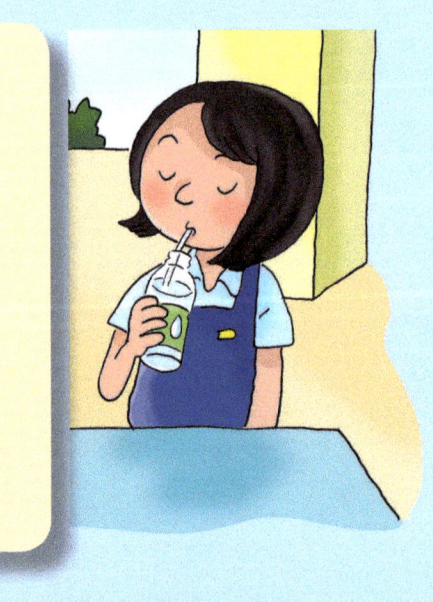

Name: Class: Date: Lesson 3

Find Your Balance

To stay healthy, you need to find a balance between the amount of food you eat and the physical activity you do.

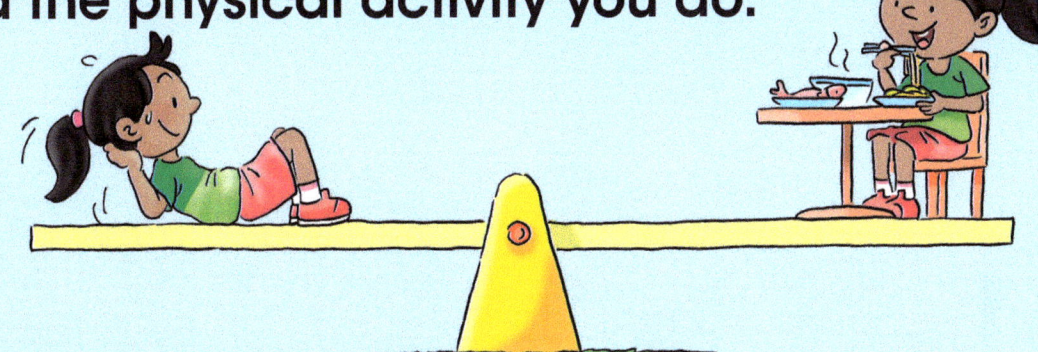

Young people who play sports or exercise daily need more food. Those who are less active or spend most of their time in front of the computer need less food.

What are some things you can do to stay healthy? List them in the space below.

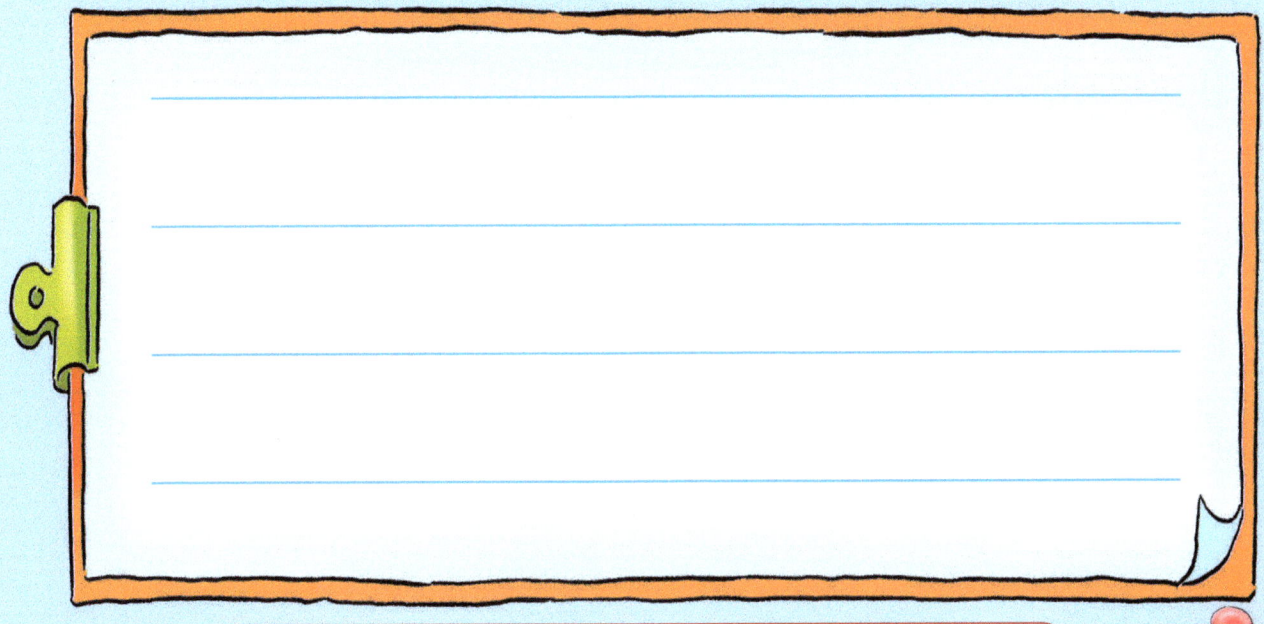

Learning Objective: Pupils will be able to understand how to achieve healthy growth.

Look at the picture below. Circle the people who are exercising or playing a sport.

Too much sitting is bad for you. You may lose concentration or start having back pain. After sitting for 30 minutes, stand up, stretch and move about.

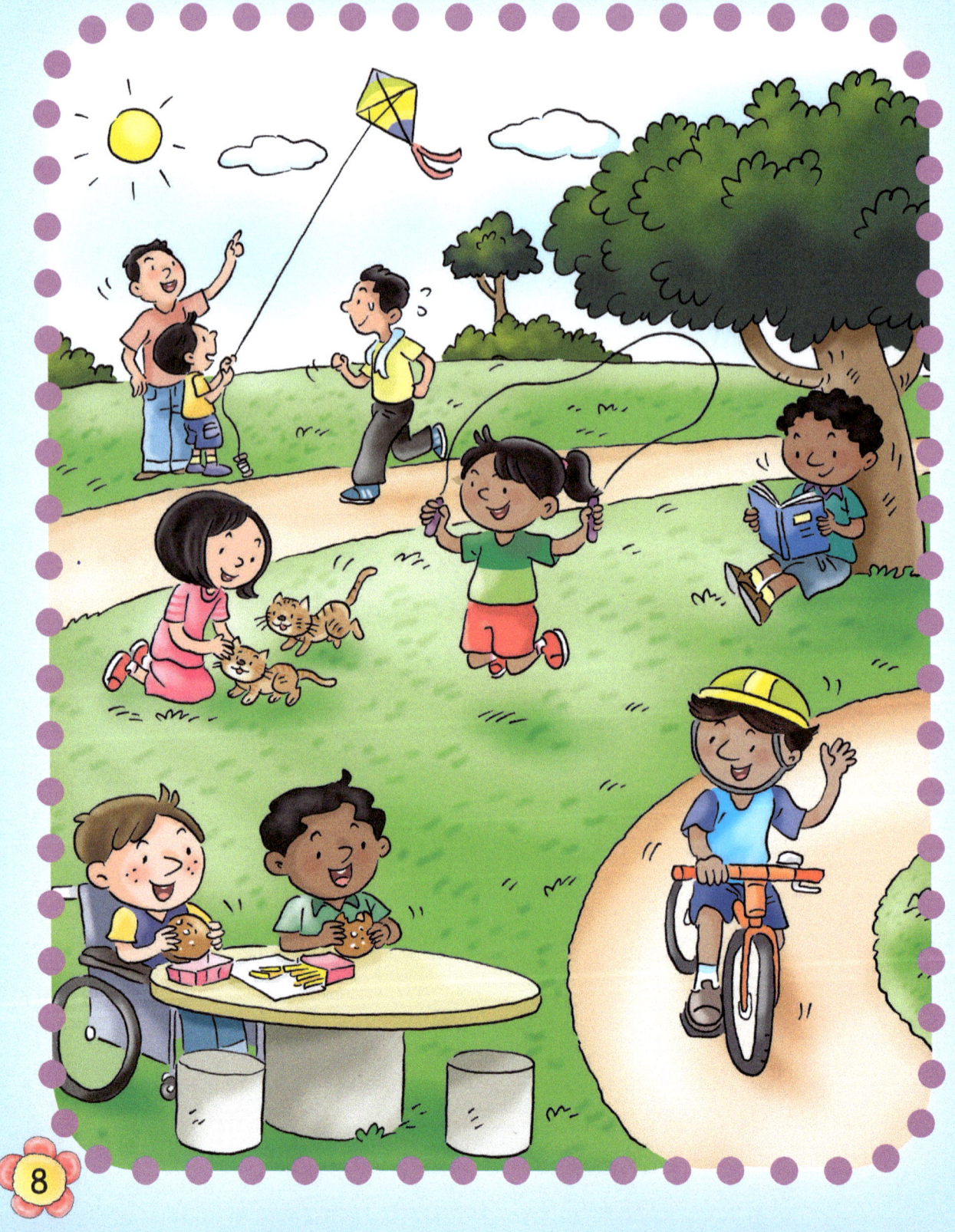

Name: Class: Date: Lesson 4

Snack Attack!

Read what the superfriends are saying.

What would you do if you get hungry between meals?

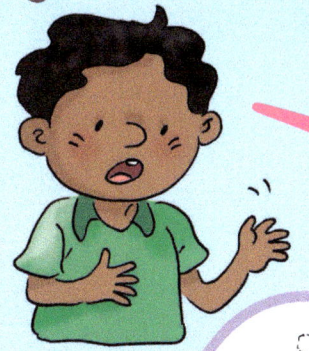

Eat, of course!

I would look for my favourite snacks – potato chips, chicken nuggets and chocolates.

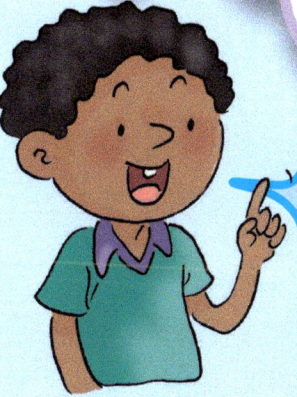

That's not very healthy. You should have something that is less sweet, salty and fatty.

And something that is not fried or processed!

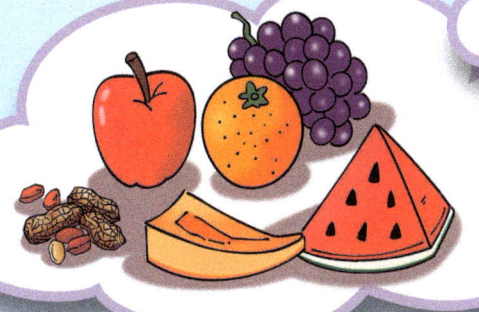

Learning Objective: Pupils will be able to understand how to achieve healthy growth.

You should avoid food that contains a lot of sugar, salt and fat. Eating too much of such food can make you obese and cause health problems.

Put a cross (✗) in the box if the picture shows food that contains a lot of sugar, salt and fat.

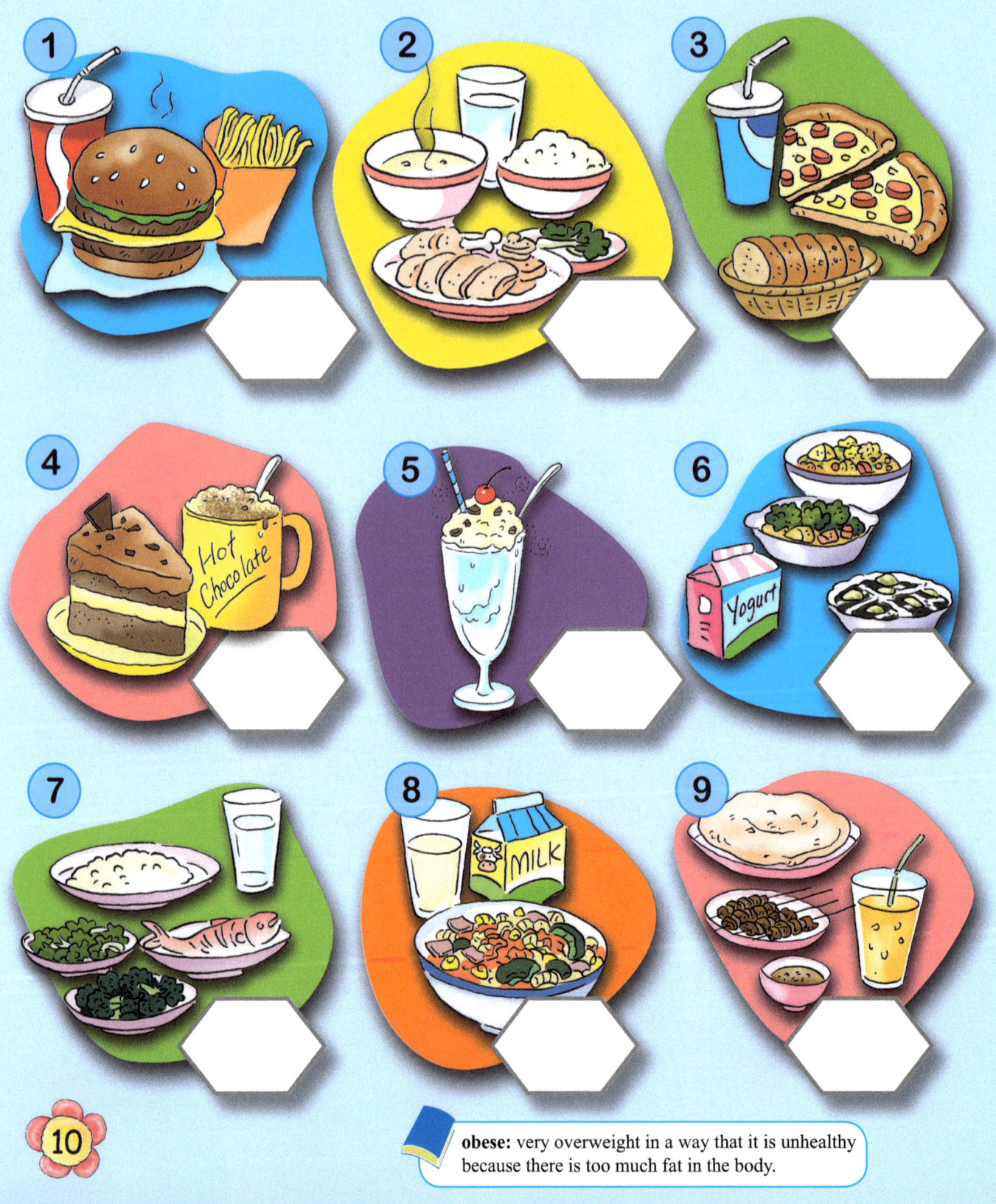

obese: very overweight in a way that it is unhealthy because there is too much fat in the body.

Name: Class: Date: Lesson 5

Fruit And Vegetables

How well do you know your fruit and vegetables? Try to solve the superfriends' riddles!

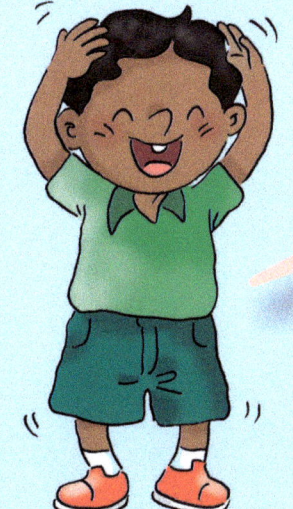

I am large and white. I have a bushy head. What am I?

c _ _ _ _ _ f _ w _ _ _

I am big and round like a ball. I am dark green on the outside but red on the inside. What am I?

_ _ t _ r _ e _ _ _ _

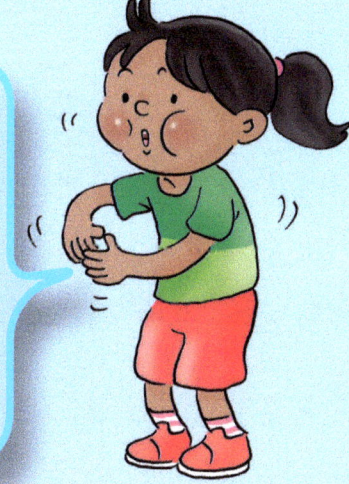

I am yellow on the outside and white on the inside. People slip when they step on my skin. What am I?

_ a _ _ n _

Learning Objective: Pupils will be able to understand how to achieve healthy growth.

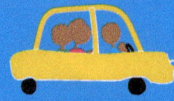 **Can you name other fruit and vegetables? Think of four examples and write them below.**

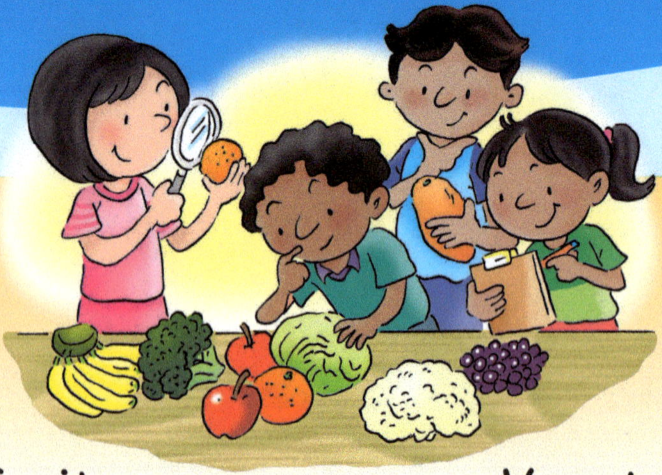

Fruit	Vegetables
_____	_____
_____	_____
_____	_____
_____	_____

To have a healthy diet, you should have at least two servings of fruit and two servings of vegetables every day.

Examples of one serving of fruit:

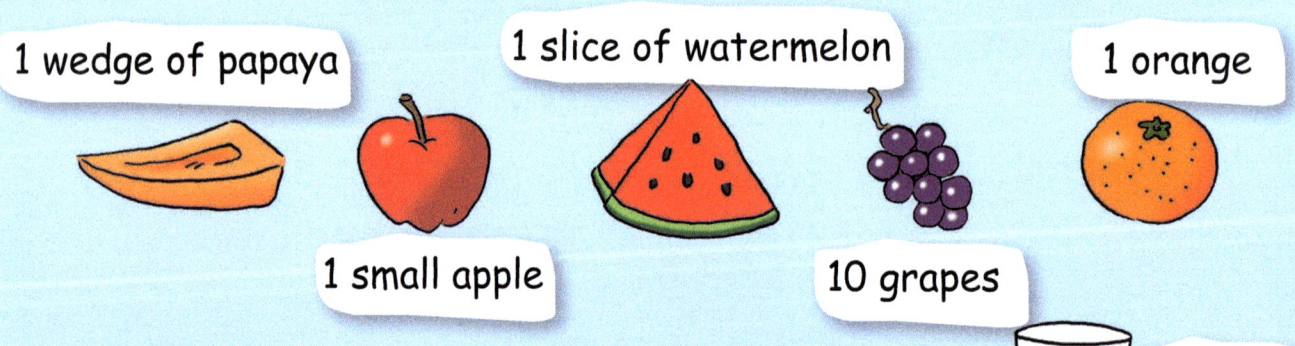

1 wedge of papaya   1 slice of watermelon   1 orange
1 small apple   10 grapes

An example of one serving of vegetables: 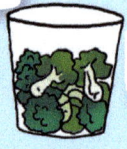 ¾ mug

Name: ⬜ Class: ⬜ Date: ⬜ Lesson 6

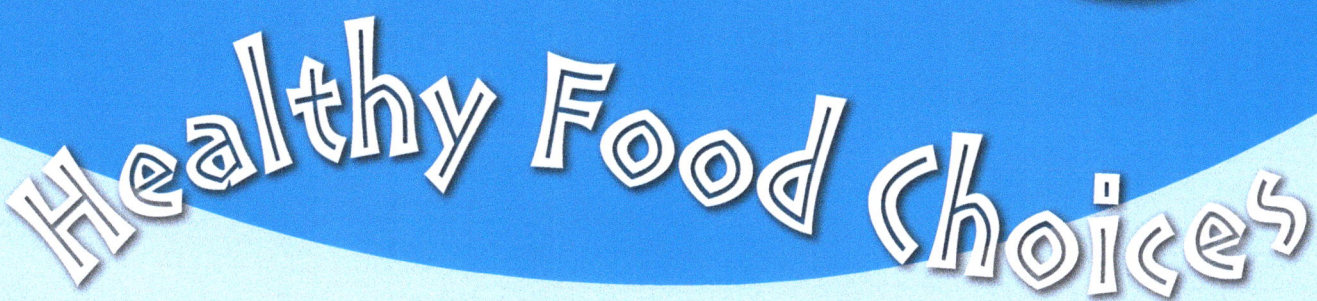

List down what you ate and drank yesterday.

Breakfast	Lunch

Dinner	Snack

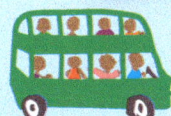

Check with the class:
- Which is the most popular meal?
- Which is the most popular snack?
- What is their favourite drink?
- Who had the earliest and latest breakfast, lunch and dinner?

Learning Objective: Pupils will be able to understand how to achieve healthy growth.

Read the statements below. Which of them describe you? Put a tick (✓) in the boxes. Then count the number of statements you have ticked.

1. I eat different types of food. ☐

2. I have three meals every day. ☐

3. I do not eat junk food. ☐

4. I snack on healthy food when I am hungry between meals. ☐

5. I eat at least two servings of fruit and vegetables every day. ☐

6. I drink at least eight glasses of water every day. ☐

If you have ticked ...

6 statements:	Well done! Keep it up!
4 to 5 statements:	You are doing quite well but you should try to improve your diet.
0 to 3 statements:	Oh no! You need to make some changes to your diet.

Name: Class: Date: **Lesson 7**

Eyes, Ears And Nose

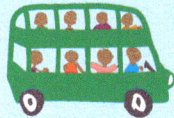 **Follow the story in the comic strip below.**

1.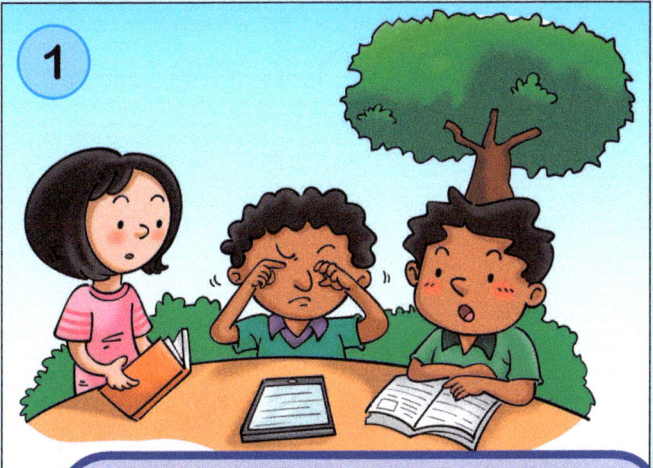

2. "What is wrong with your eyes, Ajit?"

3. "Have you been looking at the screen without any break again?"

4. "The game was too exciting. I could not stop playing!"

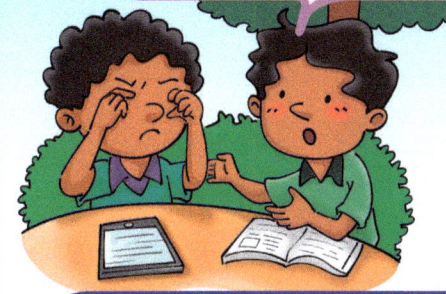

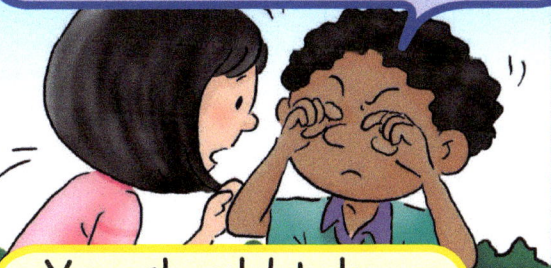

5. "You should take a break every half an hour. Get up and stretch a bit."

6. "Try looking at something in the distance. You really should spend more time outdoors too."

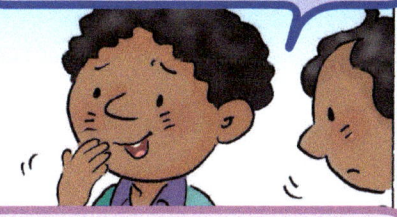

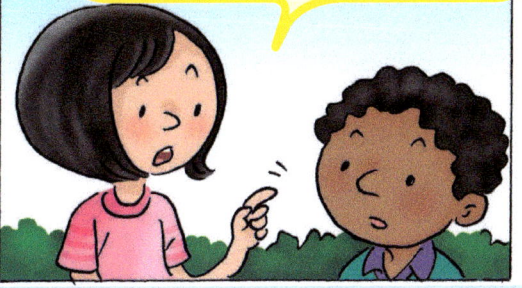

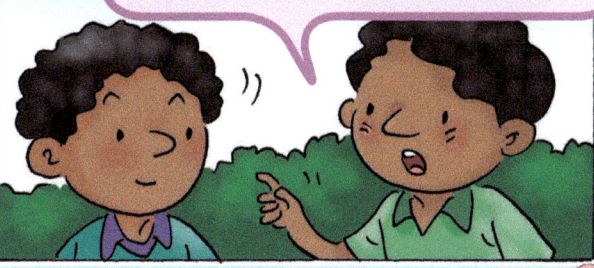

Learning Objective: Pupils will be able to establish daily habits for caring for their bodies in order to maintain or improve health and prevent illnesses.

15

Your eyes are important because they help you see. Imagine what it would be like if you cannot see anything.

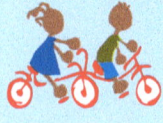 What advice did Haris and Eileen give Ajit on caring for his eyes?
Write what they said in the space below.

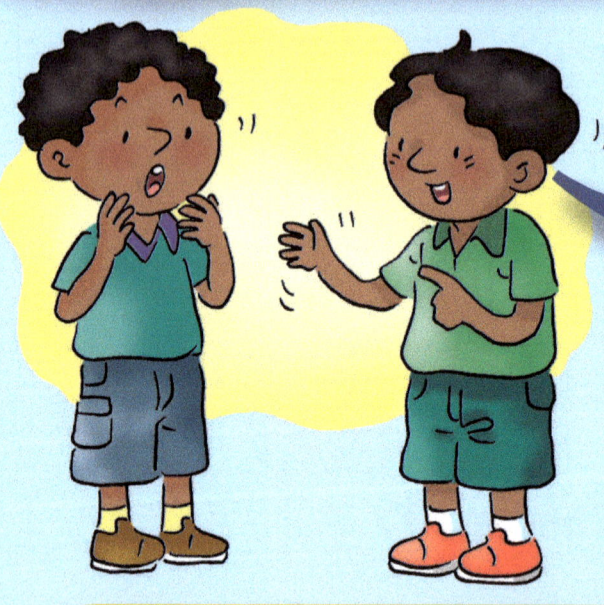

Your ears are important too. Always wipe both ears dry after a shower or a swim.

Keep your nose clean. Blow your nose gently when you have a cold. Throw the used tissue into a bin.

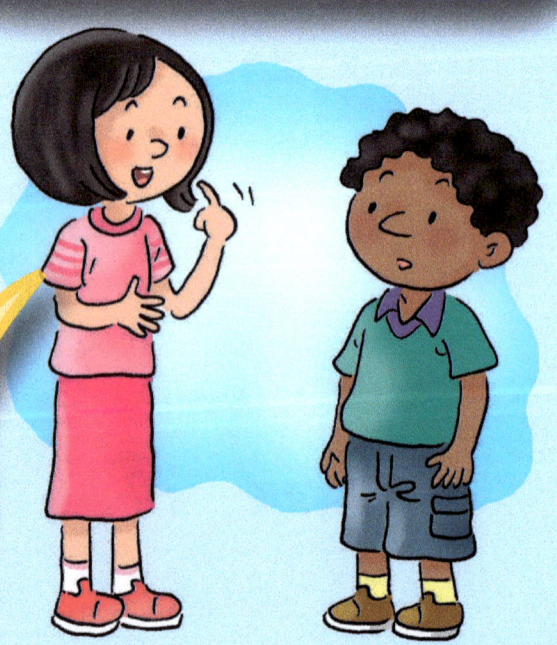

Name: Class: Date: Lesson 8

Sleep Well And Learn Better

Follow the story in the comic strip below.

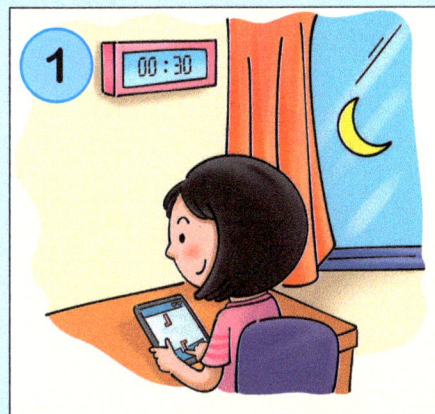
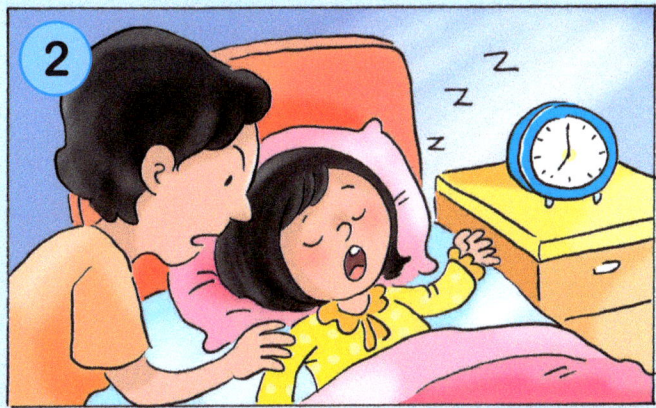
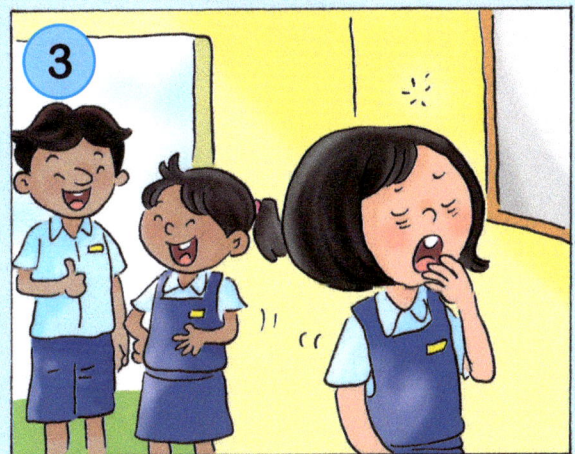
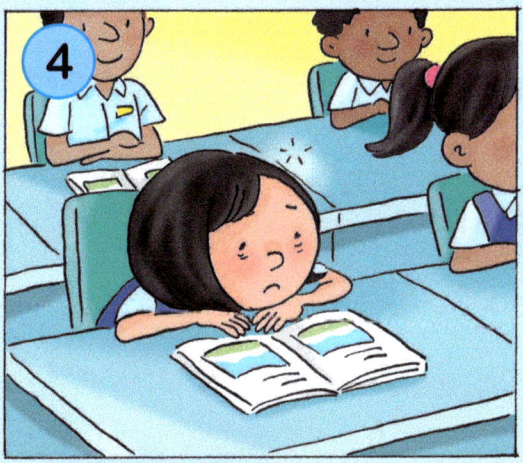
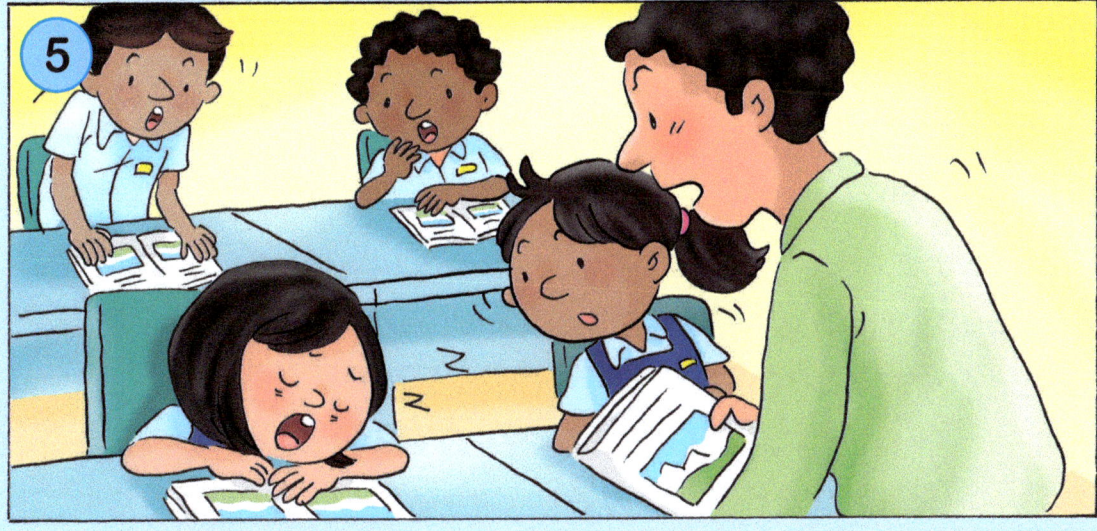

Learning Objective: Pupils will be able to establish daily habits for caring for their bodies in order to maintain or improve health and prevent illnesses.

When you sleep, your body gets a good rest. Sleep also helps you build up energy for the next day.

Look at the picture below. Colour the things that can help you sleep well.

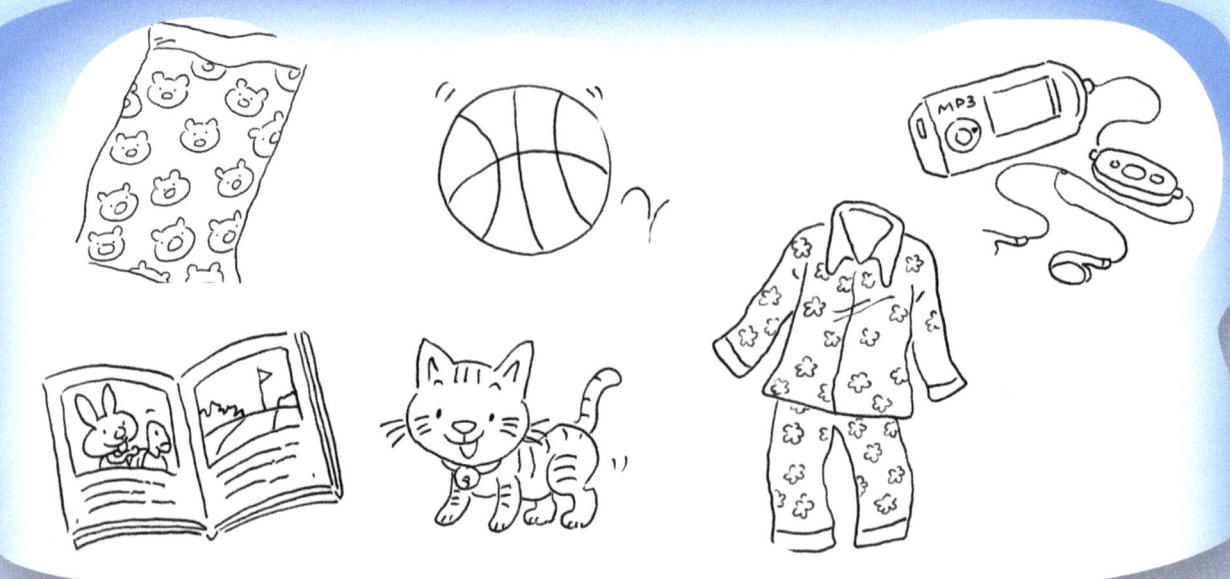

How can you get a good night's sleep?

1. Make sure the room is dark and keep it cool and well-ventilated.

2. Go to bed and wake up at the same time every day.

3. Avoid strenuous exercises four hours before bedtime.

4. Sleep for nine to ten hours every night.

5. Do not go to bed hungry or immediately after a heavy meal.

6. Stop using electronic gadgets and watching TV one hour before bedtime.

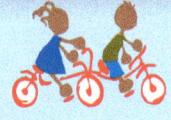 What happens when you do not have enough sleep?

Name: Class: Date: Lesson 9

Stop Spreading Germs

Follow the story in the comic strip below. What did the superfriends do wrongly and what happened as a result?

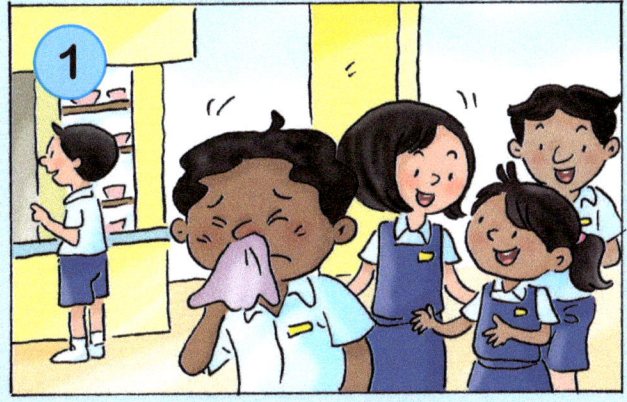
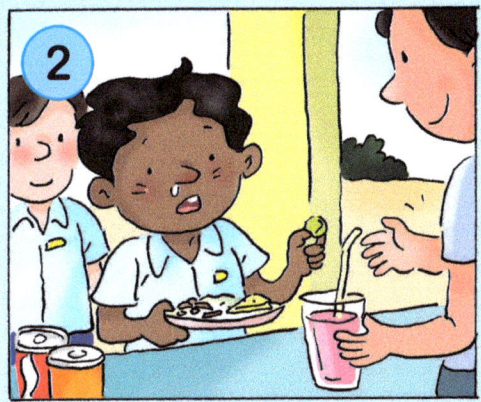
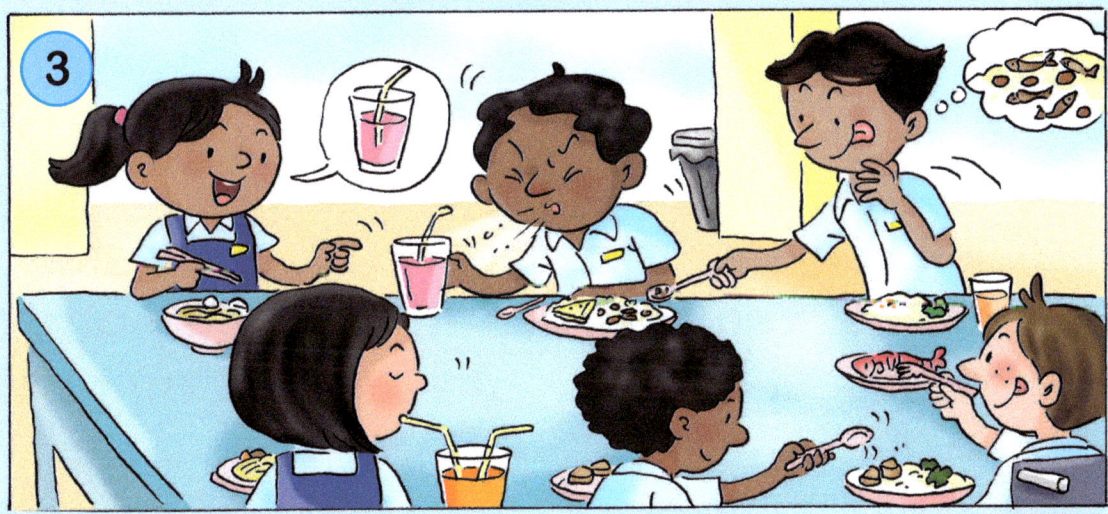
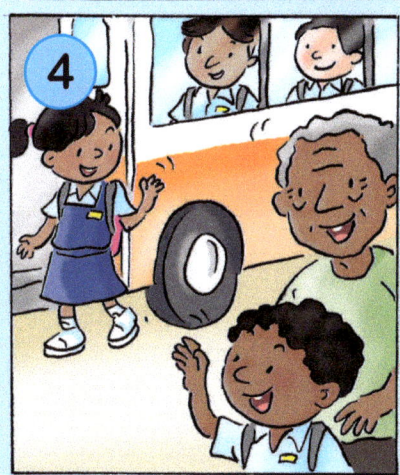
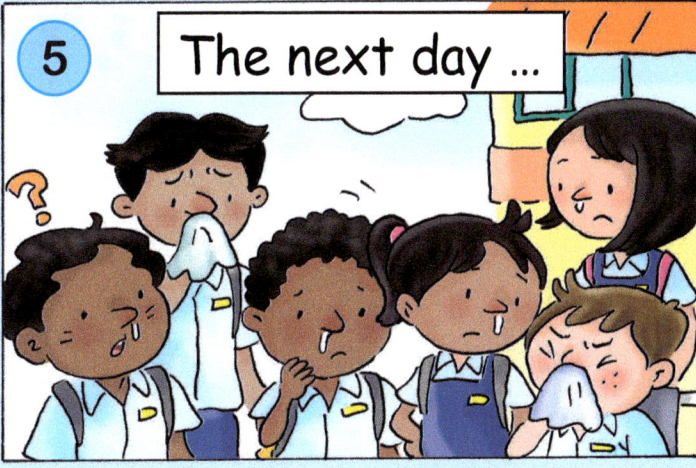

The next day …

Learning Objective: Pupils will be able to establish daily habits for caring for their bodies in order to maintain or improve health and prevent illnesses.

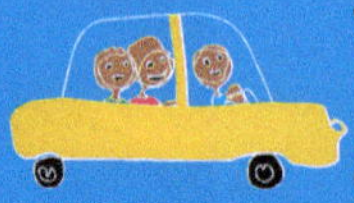

You are infectious when you have a cough or cold. List five things you could do to stop the spread of germs.

1. 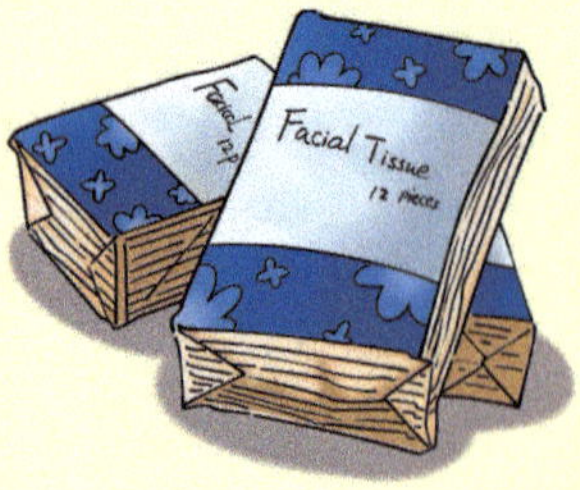
2. 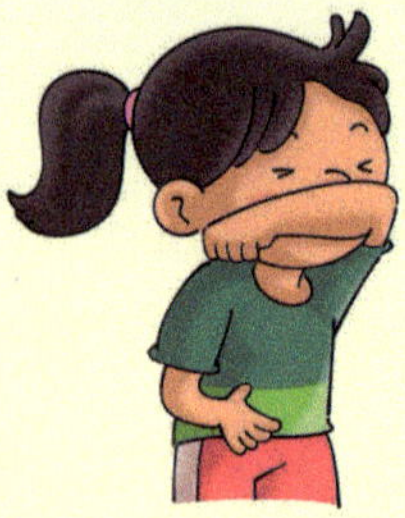
3. 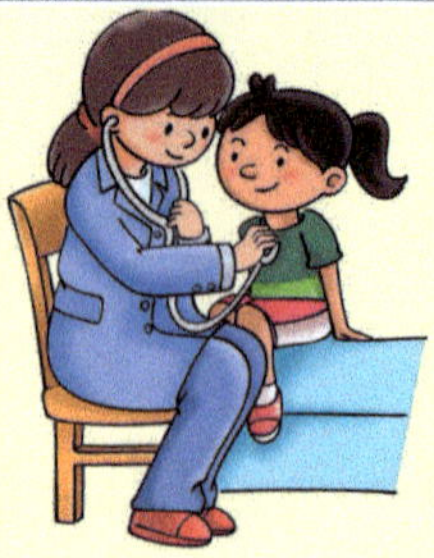
4. 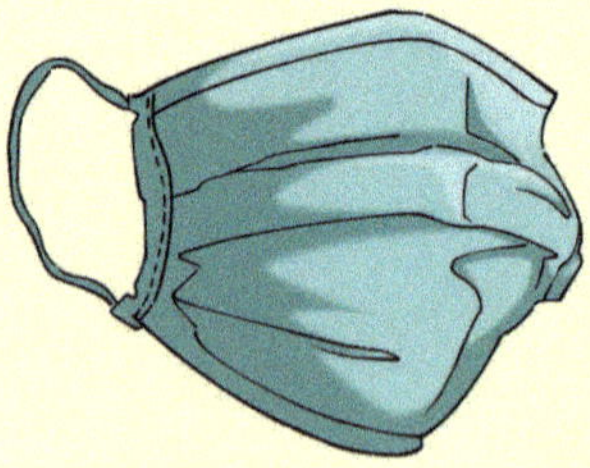
5.

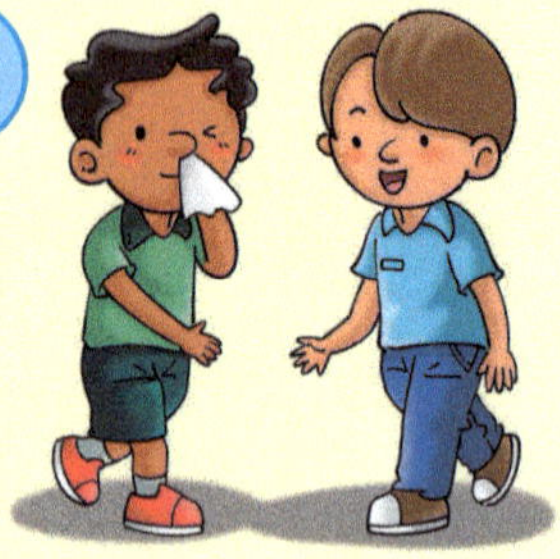

Remember: wash your hands before and after meals, after using the toilet, after exercise and sport, and after you get home from school or an outing.

Seven Steps To Hand Hygiene

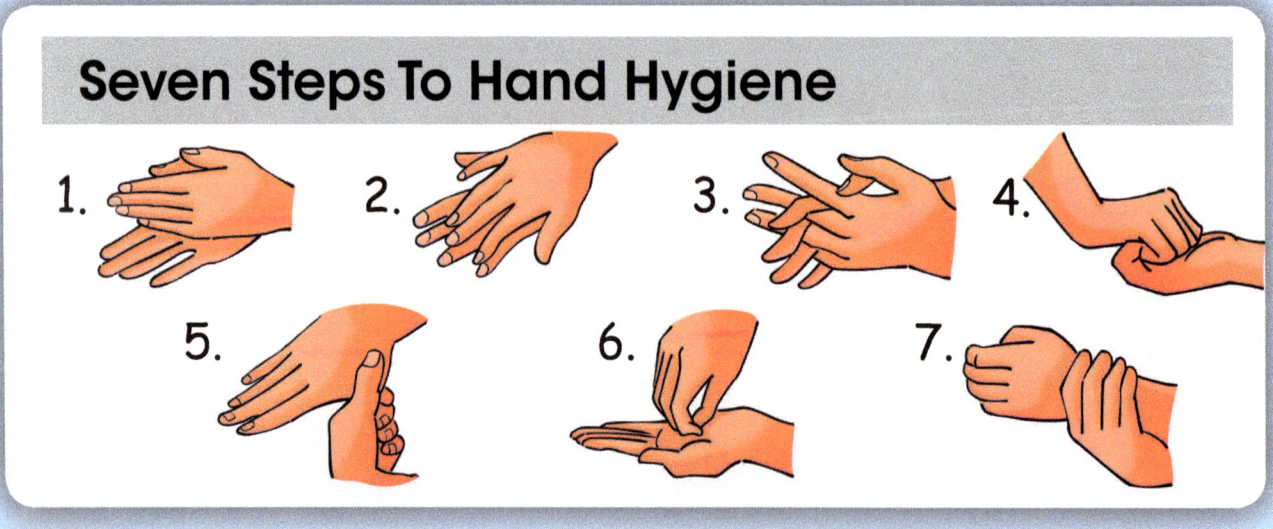

1.
2.
3.
4.
5.
6.
7.

Name: ___ Class: ___ Date: ___

Lesson 10

Gums, Teeth And Tongue

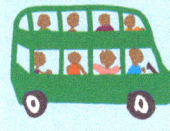 Harold, Lam and Haris are at an exhibition about animals. Read what they are saying.

Wow! Look at how sharp the shark's teeth are!

Shark's teeth

That is because they need to tear their food apart.

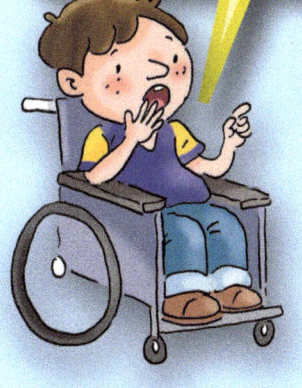

Camel's teeth

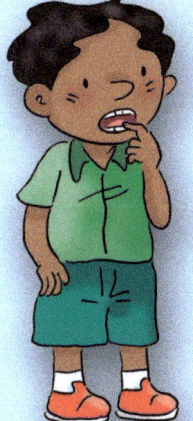 **See how different the camel's teeth are. I wonder why they are shaped like that.**

Learning Objective: Pupils will be able to recognise the importance of developing good oral hygiene habits to ensure that the teeth are healthy and well maintained.

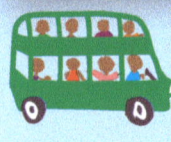 Open your mouth and look into a mirror. What different shapes of teeth do you see? Draw them in the space below.

 Unlike animals, you do not just use your teeth for eating. You need your teeth and tongue to speak well.

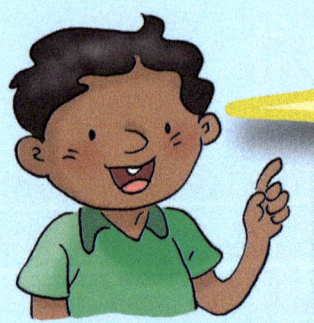 Try saying this without using your tongue to touch your teeth. "Tell the tall doctor my brother has pain in his lower teeth!"

Your tongue helps you taste your food too. What can food taste like?

S _ _ R   _P_CY   S _ _ TY

B _ _ TE _   _WE_T

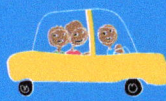 **Read each sentence below. Circle 'T' if it is true and 'F' if it is false.**

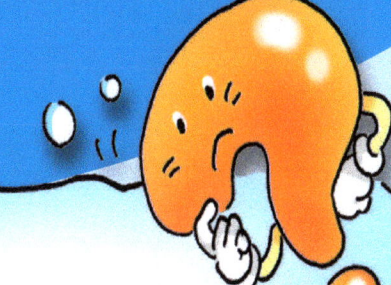

1. My gums hold my teeth in place. T/F

2. Keeping my teeth and tongue clean will prevent tooth decay and bad breath. T/F

3. I will have three sets of teeth in my lifetime. T/F

4. I need teeth to chew my food. T/F

5. My tongue helps me taste the food. T/F

6. Brushing my teeth and tongue once a day will help keep them clean. T/F

7. You should use a lot of toothpaste when brushing your teeth. T/F

8. When I lose a milk tooth, a permanent tooth will grow at the same place. T/F

9. I should rinse my mouth after eating. T/F

Learning Objective: Pupils will be able to recognise the importance of developing good oral hygiene habits to ensure that the teeth are healthy and well maintained.

There are things you can use to keep your mouth clean. Circle them in the maze below. Then draw a line to connect them from 'start' to 'end'.

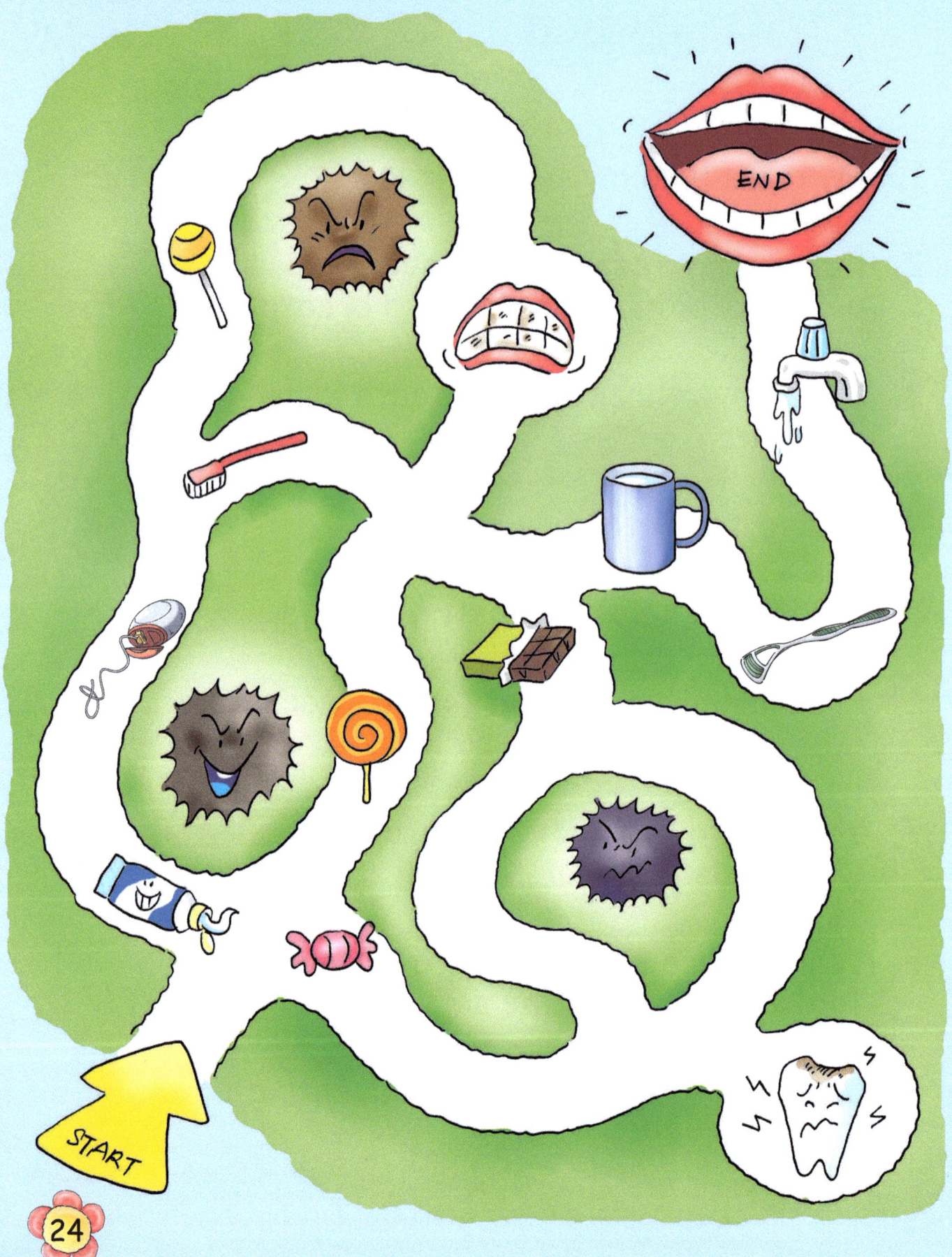

Lesson 11

Brush Your Teeth And Gums

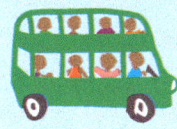 Sing the song below.

Brush your teeth and gums
Brush them every day.
Once in the morning, once in the evening,
Clear the plaque away!

Floss, floss, floss your teeth
Floss them every day.
Once in the morning, once in the evening,
Flick the bits away!

Scrape, scrape, scrape your tongue
Scrape it every day.
Once in the morning, once in the evening,
Scrape the germs away!

Learning Objective: Pupils will be able to recognise the importance of developing good oral hygiene habits to ensure that the teeth are healthy and well-maintained.

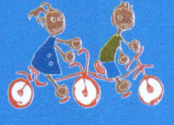 Exchange your Pupil's Books with your partner. Brush your gums, teeth and tongue in front of him or her. Your partner will give you a score from 1 to 10.

/10

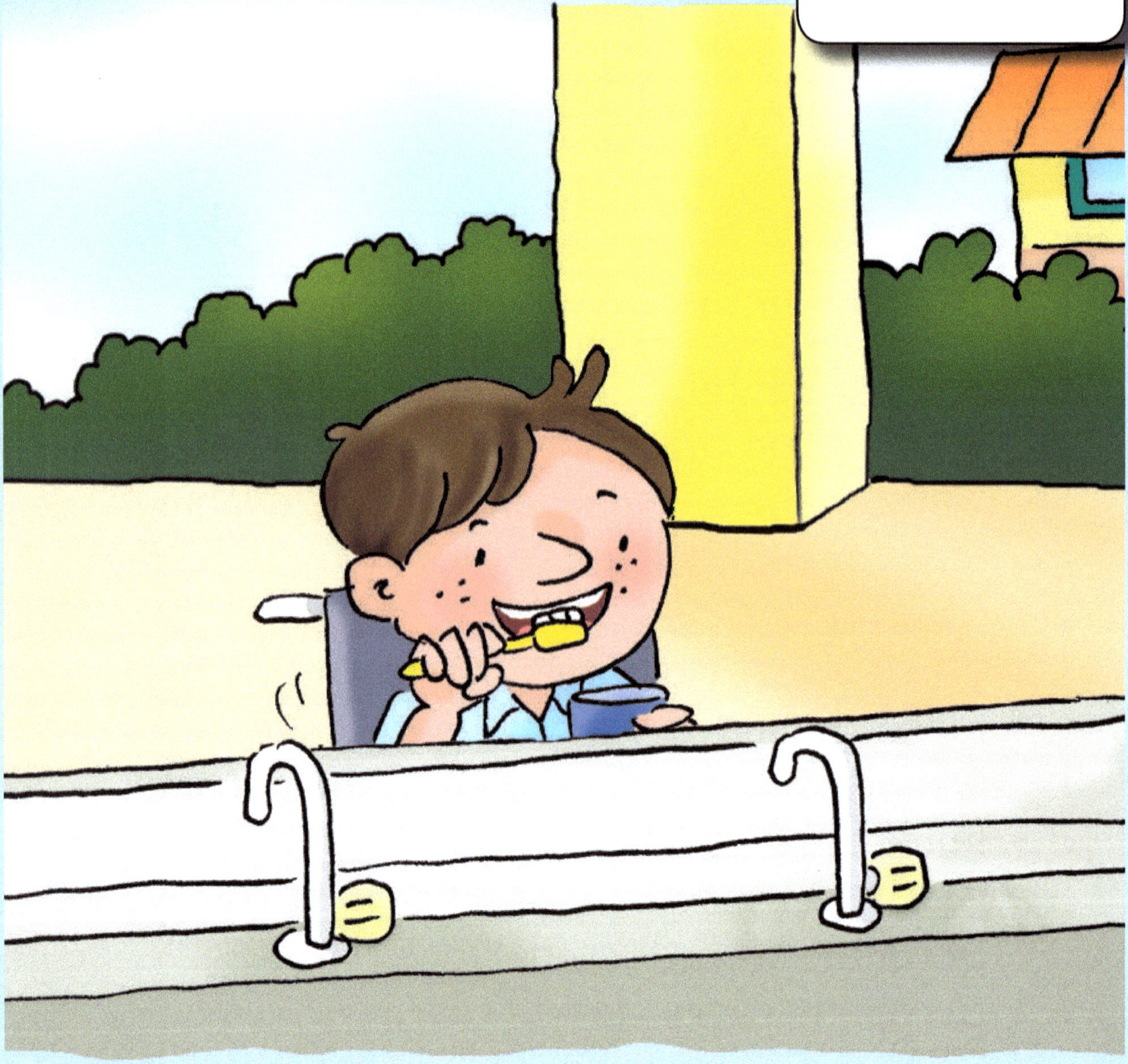

If you scored ...

9 – 10: Well done!

6 – 8: You are doing quite well. Keep it up!

1 – 5: Ask your partner how you can improve.

Environment And Your Health

In this section, you will learn:

- about common causes of road accidents;
- some road safety rules; and
- how to prevent germs from spreading diseases.

Name: Class: Date:

Lesson 1

Crossing Safely

The safest way to cross a road is to use a pedestrian crossing.

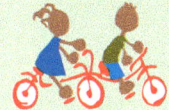 Which superfriend is using a pedestrian crossing? Put a tick (✓) in the boxes.

1.

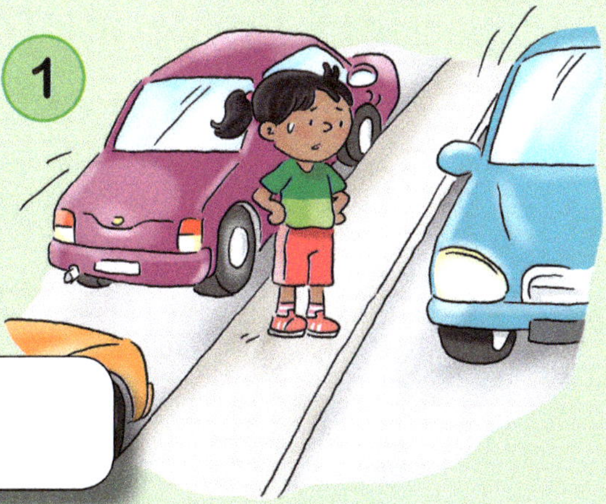

2.

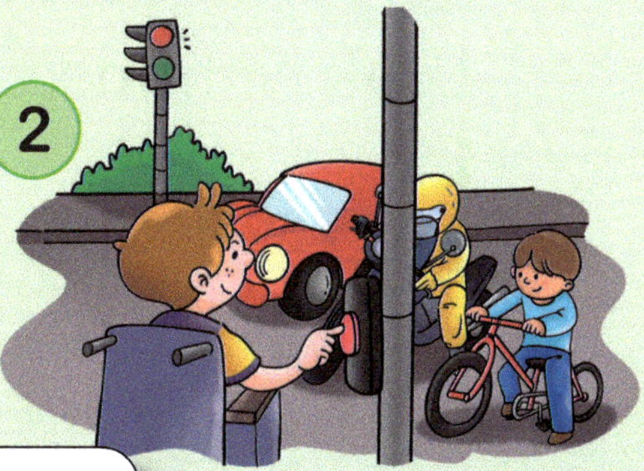

3.

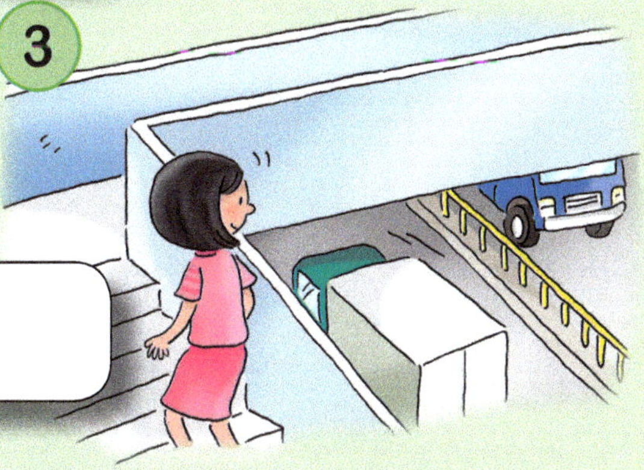

4.

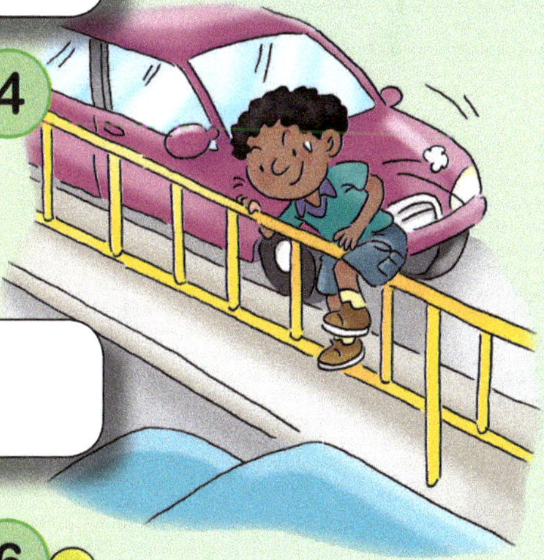

5.

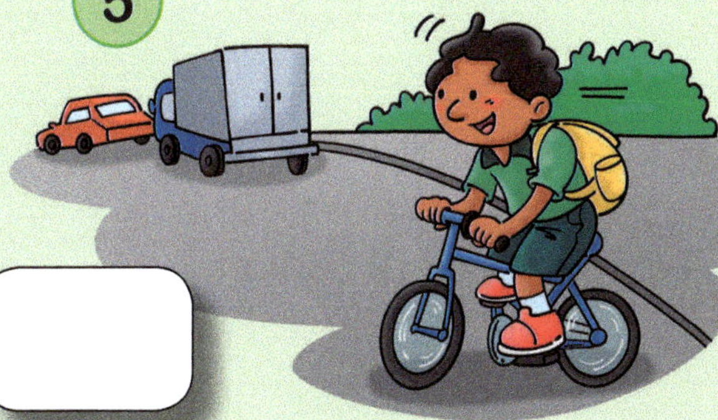

6.

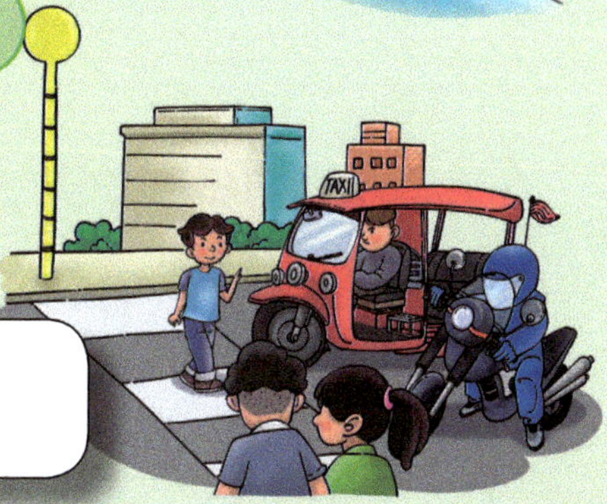

Learning Objective: Pupils will be able to understand that it is everyone's responsibility to keep safe by paying attention to environmental dangers.

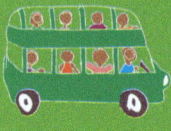 Have you heard of the kerb drill? Read the instructions and look at the pictures below. Try doing the kerb drill now!

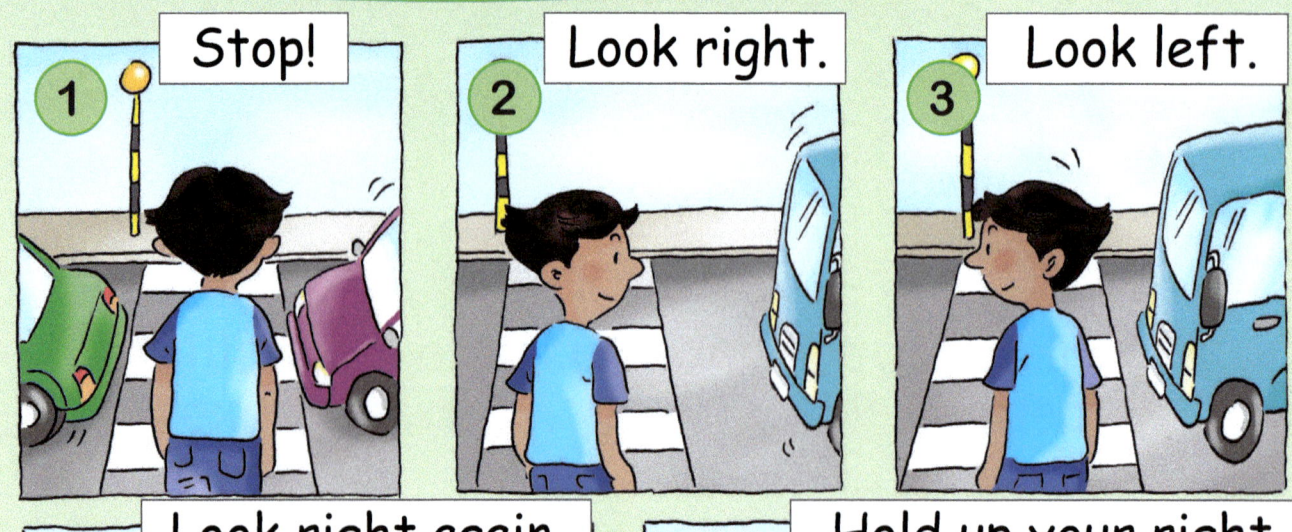

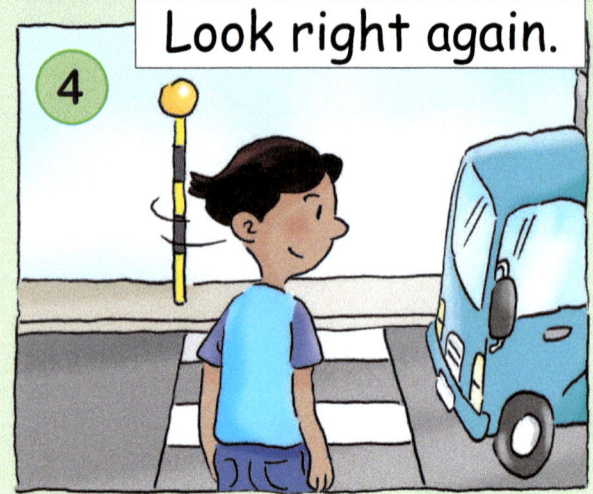

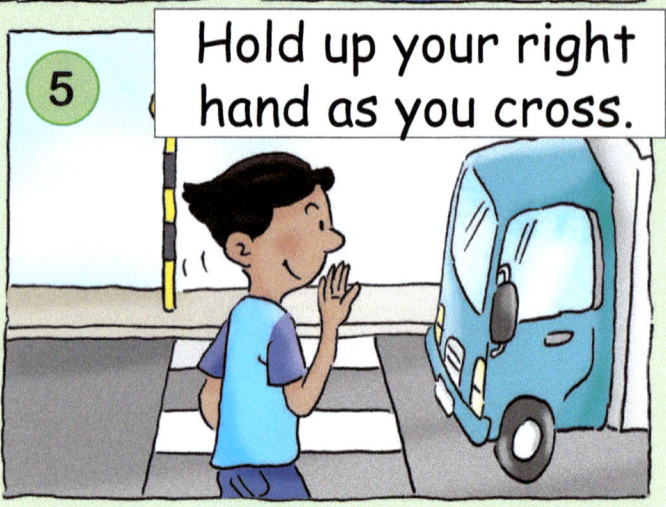

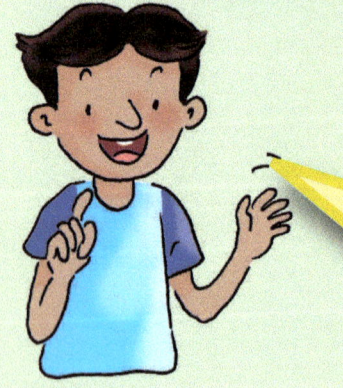 Remember to do the kerb drill whenever you cross a road at a traffic junction or use a zebra crossing.

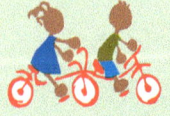 Exchange your Pupil's Book with your partner. Do the kerb drill for each other. Ask your partner to give you a score to show how well you did the drill.

/10

Name: Class: Date:

Lesson 2

What Went Wrong?

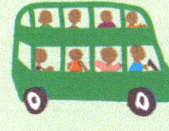

Oh no! The superfriends did not practise road safety when crossing the road. Look at the photographs Harold took of them. What is wrong in each photograph?

1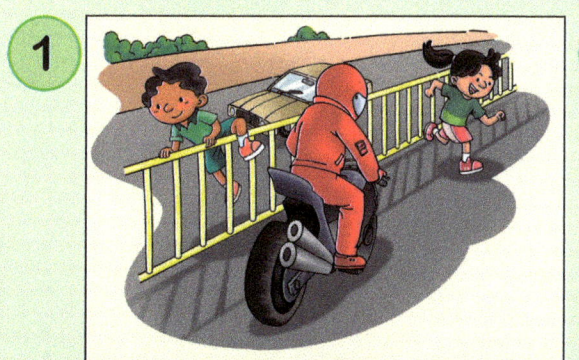

2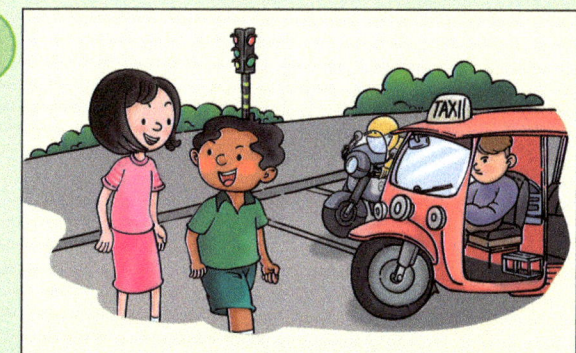

3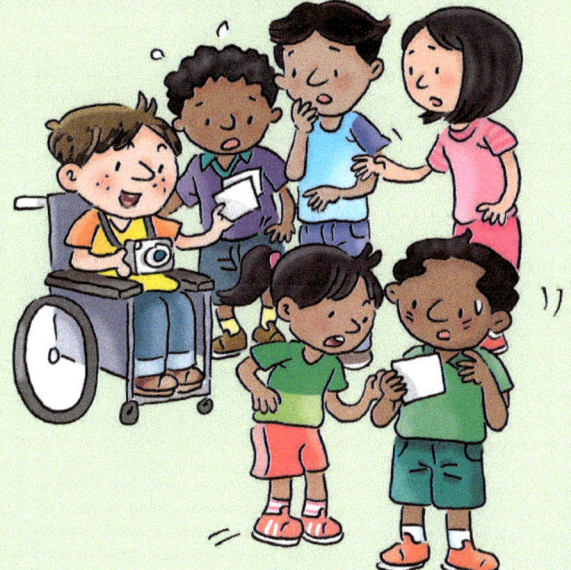

4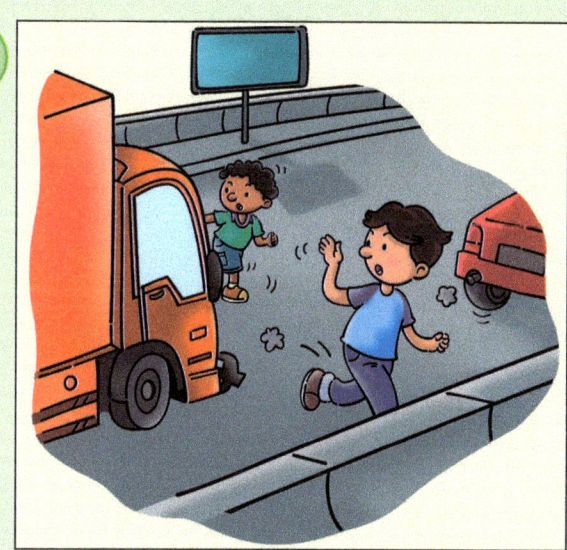

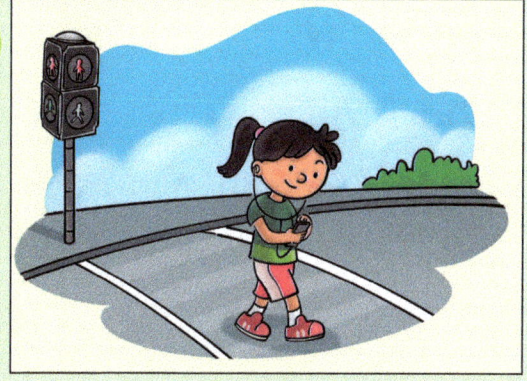

Learning Objective: Pupils will be able to understand that it is everyone's responsibility to keep safe by paying attention to environmental dangers.

Harold created the following poster to teach his friends about road safety. Fill in the blanks below.

1. Never _l_m_ or j_ _ p over road dividers.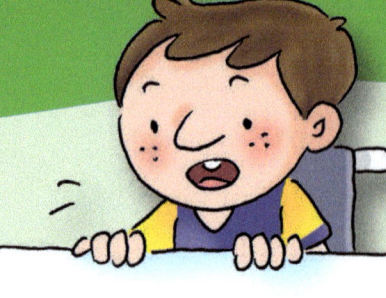

2. Always use a p_ _ _ _ s_ _ _ _ _ n crossing and pay _ _ t _ _ _ ion when crossing the road.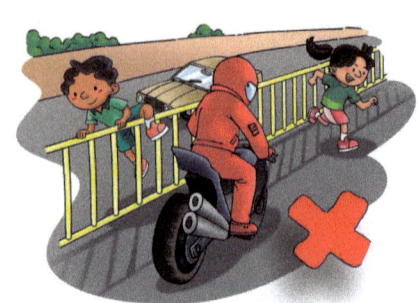

3. Never c _ _ _ s _ an expressway.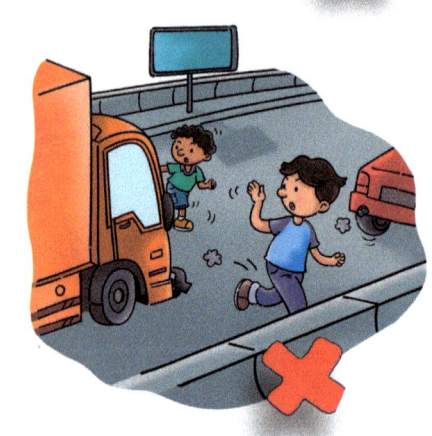

4. Do not look at your _ _ o _ e or smart device while crossing the road, even at the pedestrian crossing!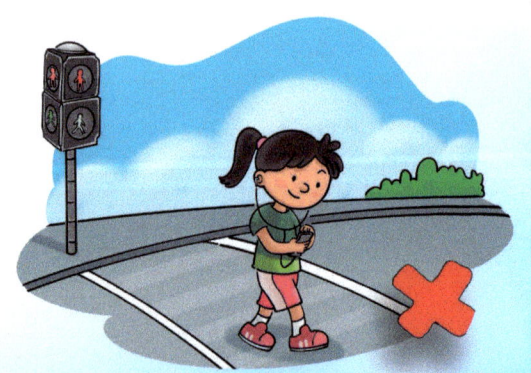

Name: Class: Date:

Safety Rules I

Look at the pictures below. What do you think the superfriends are doing incorrectly?

1

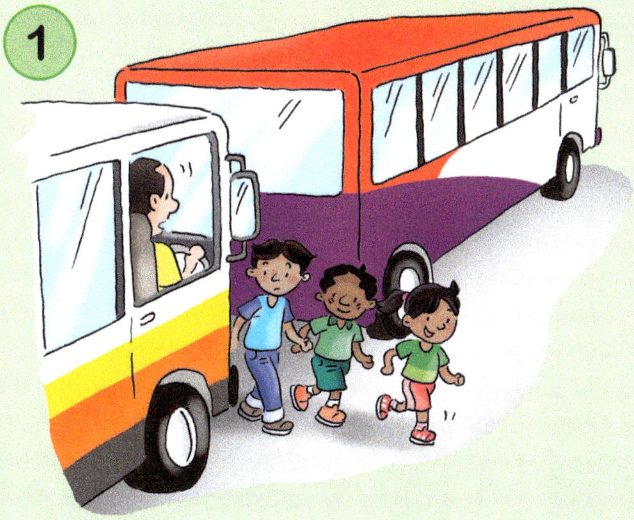

2

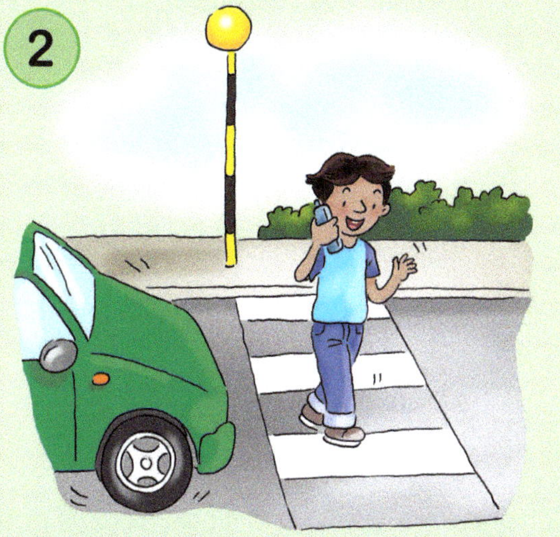

3

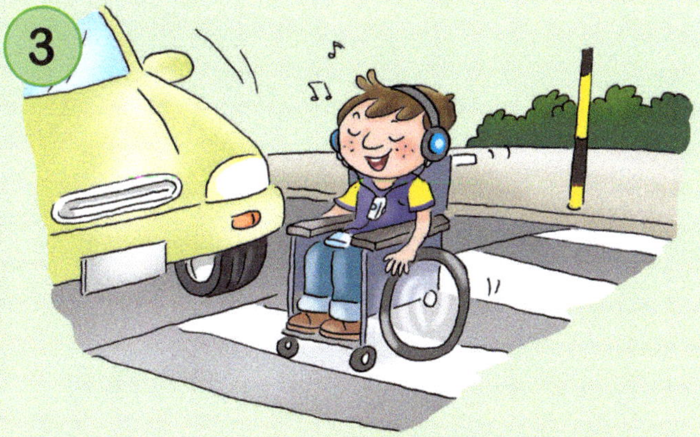

4

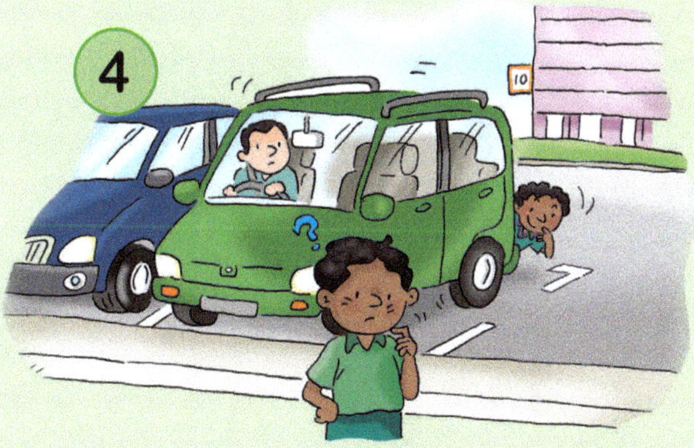

5

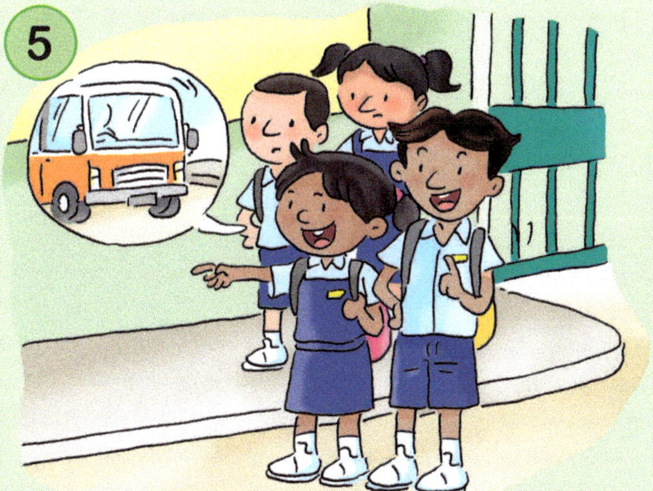

6

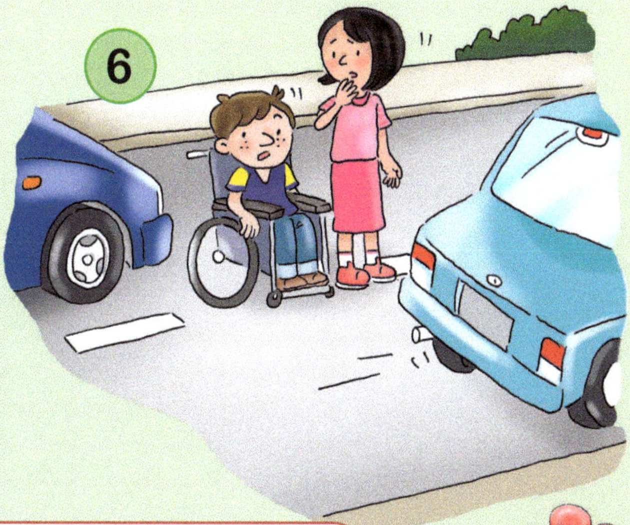

Learning Objective: Pupils will be able to understand that it is everyone's responsibility to keep safe by paying attention to environmental dangers.

It looks like there are more road safety rules than what the superfriends have already learnt.

Fill in the blanks below to find out other road safety rules. Use the pictures to help you.

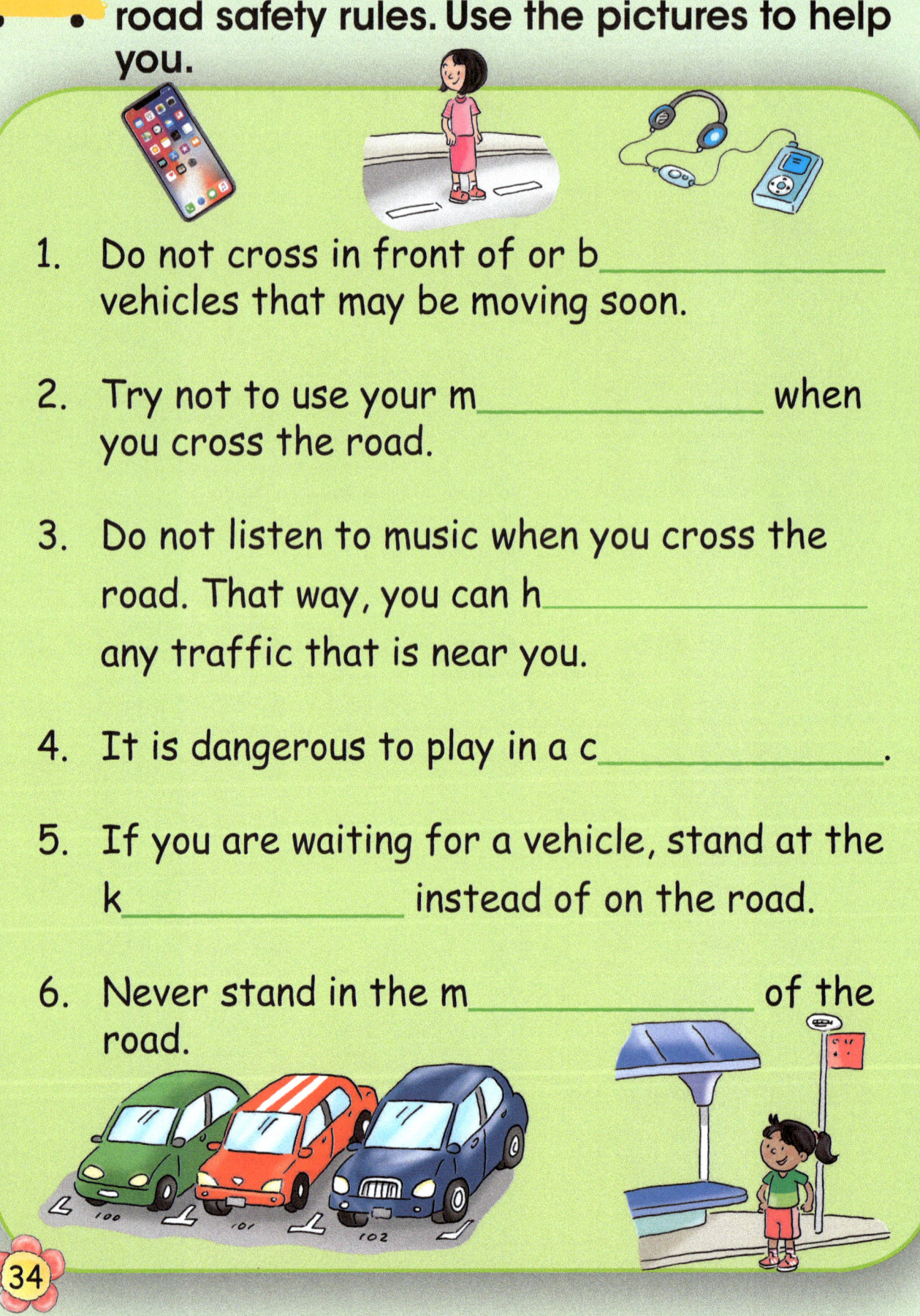

1. Do not cross in front of or b_____ vehicles that may be moving soon.

2. Try not to use your m_____ when you cross the road.

3. Do not listen to music when you cross the road. That way, you can h_____ any traffic that is near you.

4. It is dangerous to play in a c_____.

5. If you are waiting for a vehicle, stand at the k_____ instead of on the road.

6. Never stand in the m_____ of the road.

Name: Class: Date:

Lesson 4

Safety Rules II

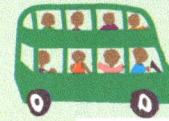 Follow the story in the comic strip below.

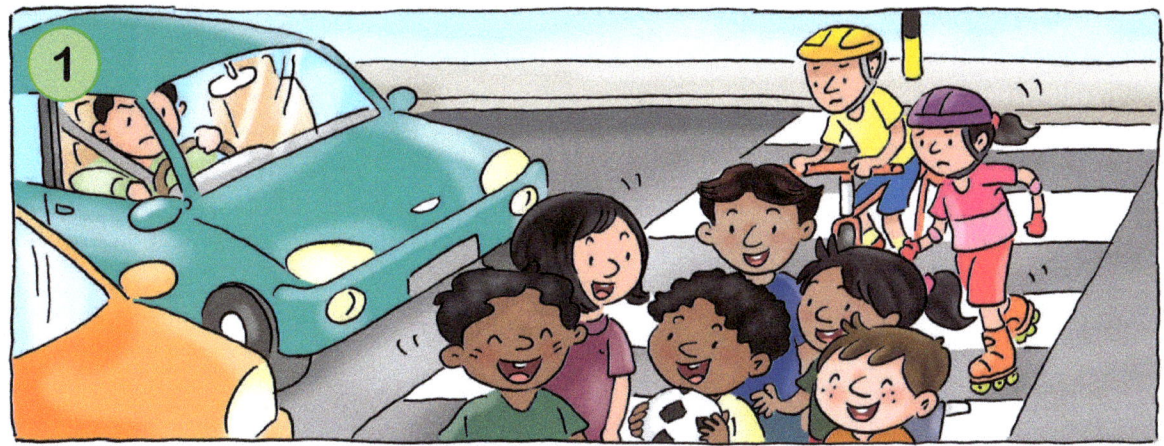

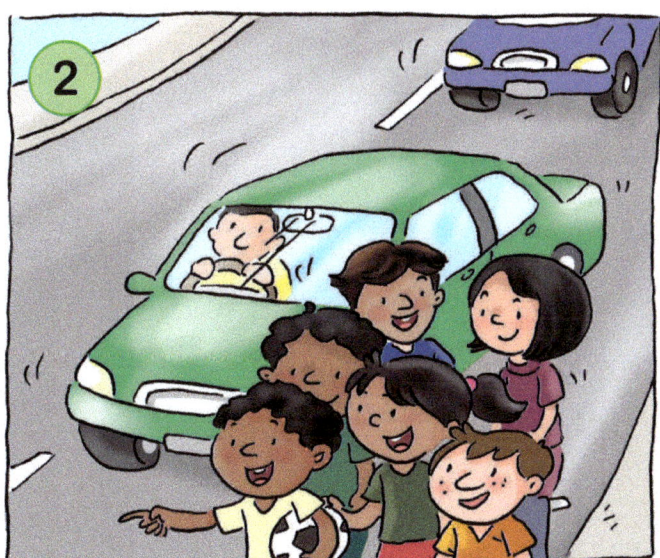

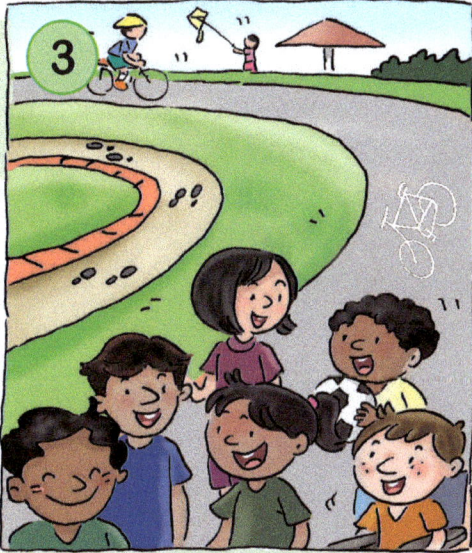

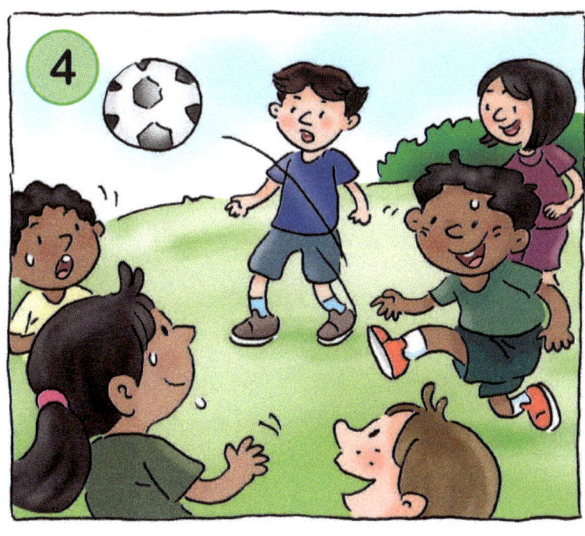

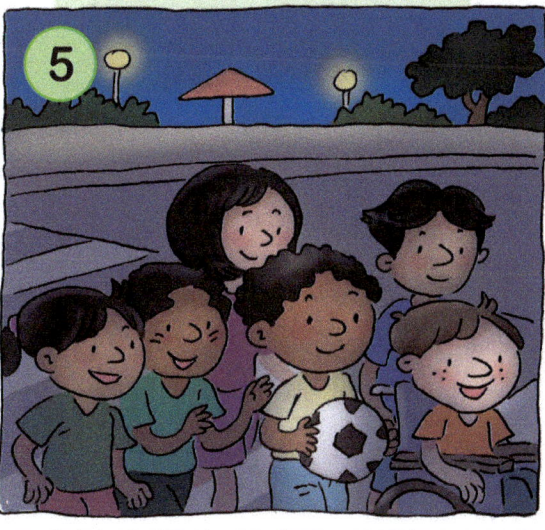

Learning Objective: Pupils will be able to understand that it is everyone's responsibility to keep safe by paying attention to environmental dangers.

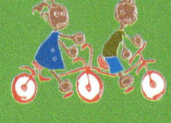 Look at the pictures. What should the superfriends have done? Join the yellow to the blue dots to form four statements.

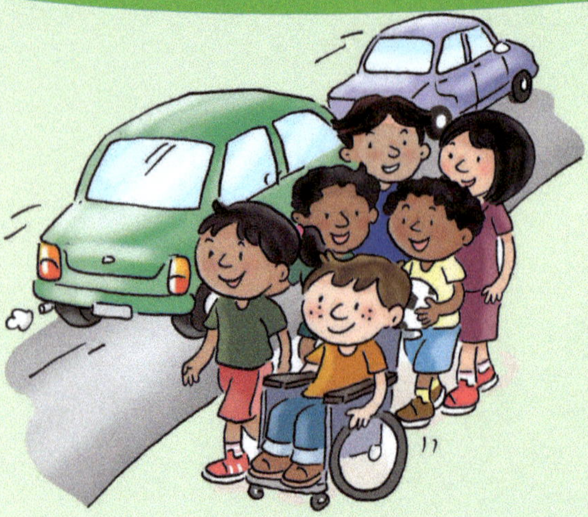

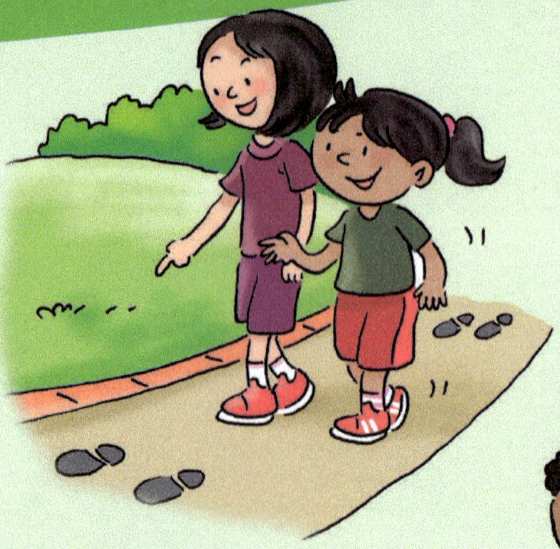

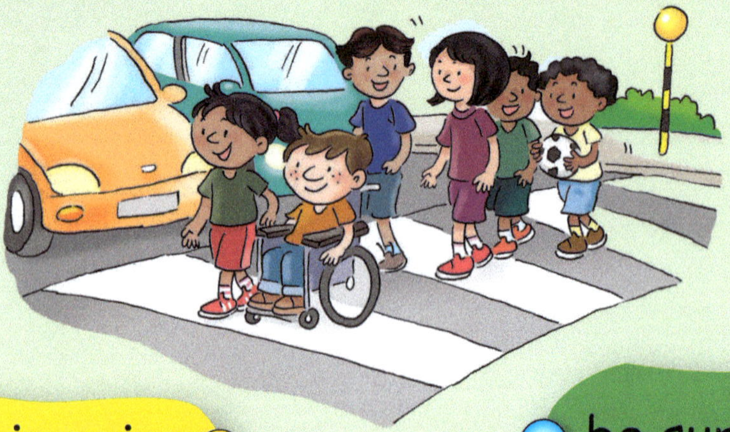

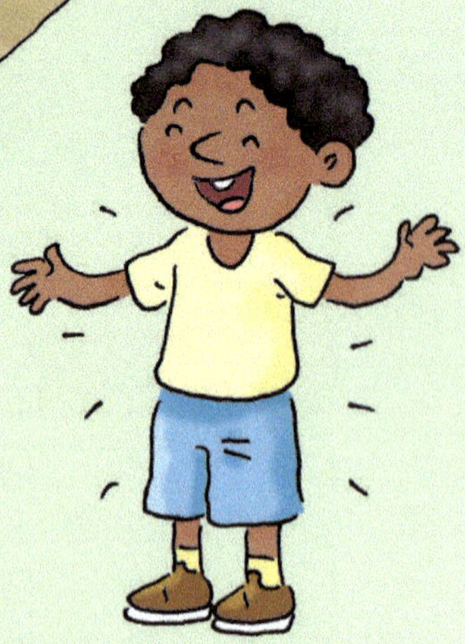

- Walk in pairs — when you are in a group.
- Always walk — on footpaths.
- If you have to walk along the road, — be sure to face the oncoming traffic
- Always wear light-coloured clothing at night — so that others can see you clearly.

Name: Class: Date:

Lessons 5 & 6

Road Safety First

🚴 **Colour the superfriends who are breaking road safety rules.**

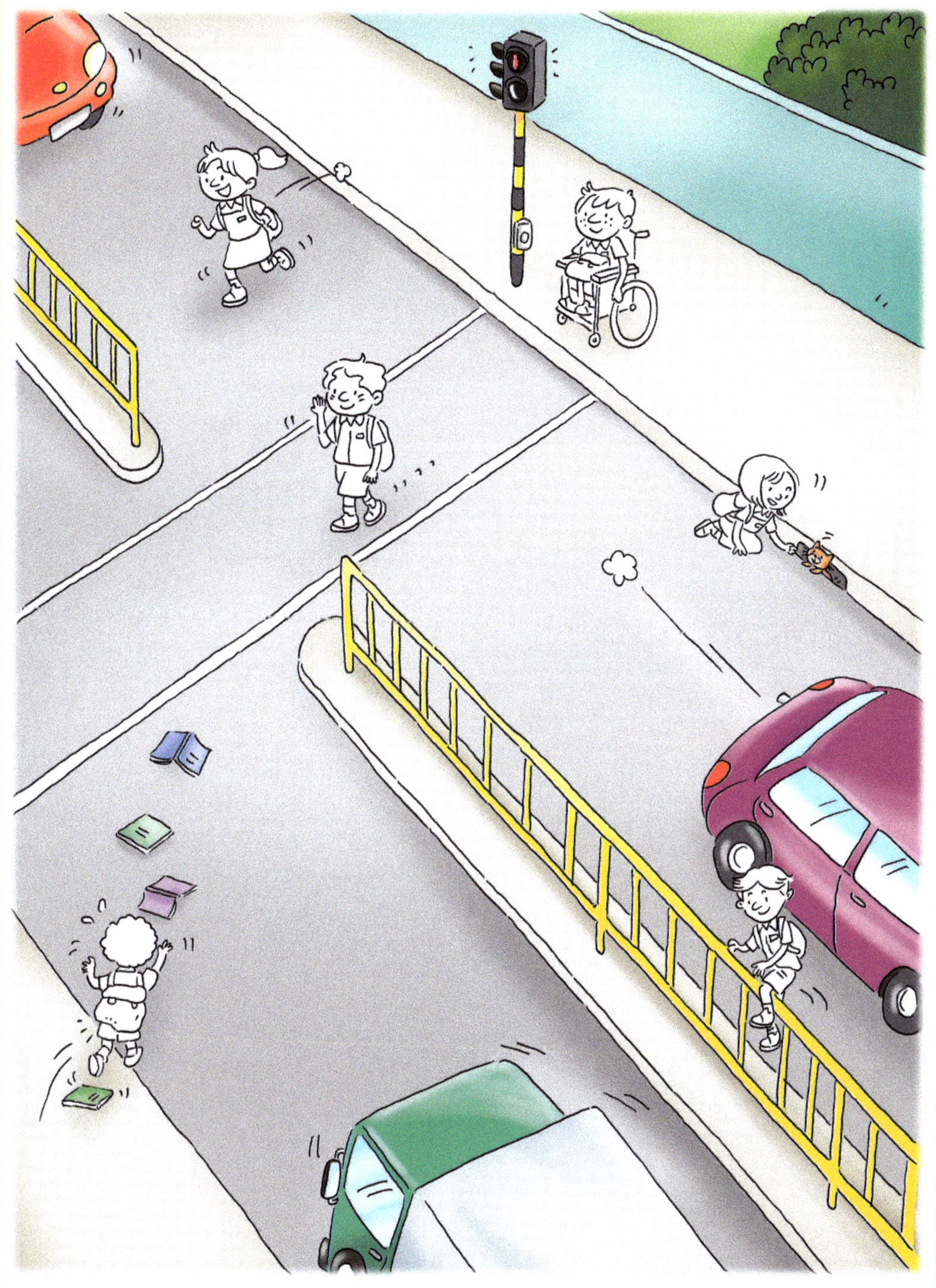

Learning Objective: Pupils will be able to understand that it is everyone's responsibility to keep safe by paying attention to environmental dangers.

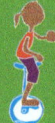 Try to remember all the road safety rules you have learnt. Which are the most important in your city?

Create your own road safety poster below. List five things you should and should not do.

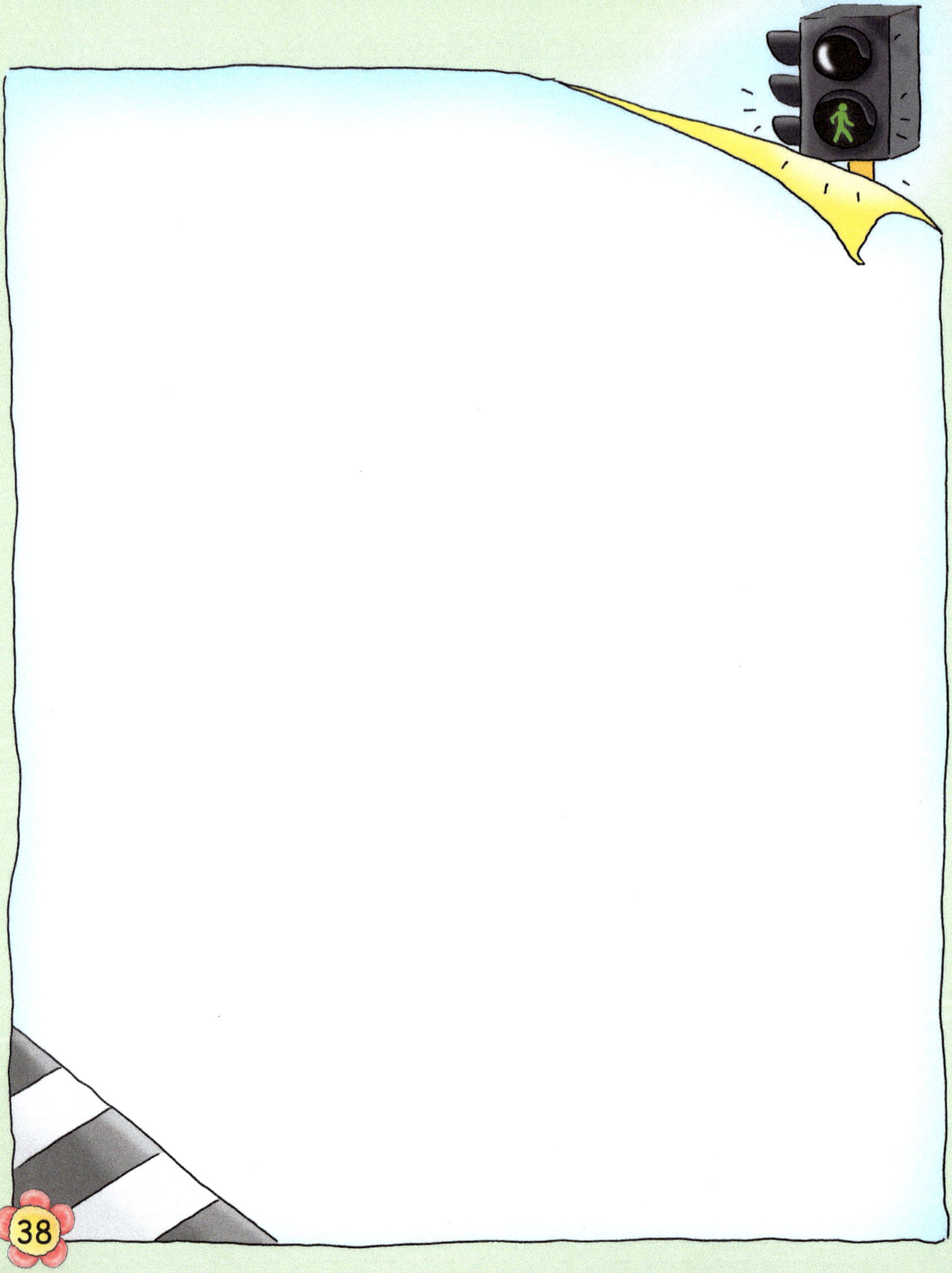

Germs Can Make You Sick

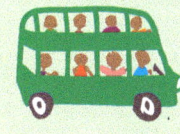

Follow the story in the comic strip below.

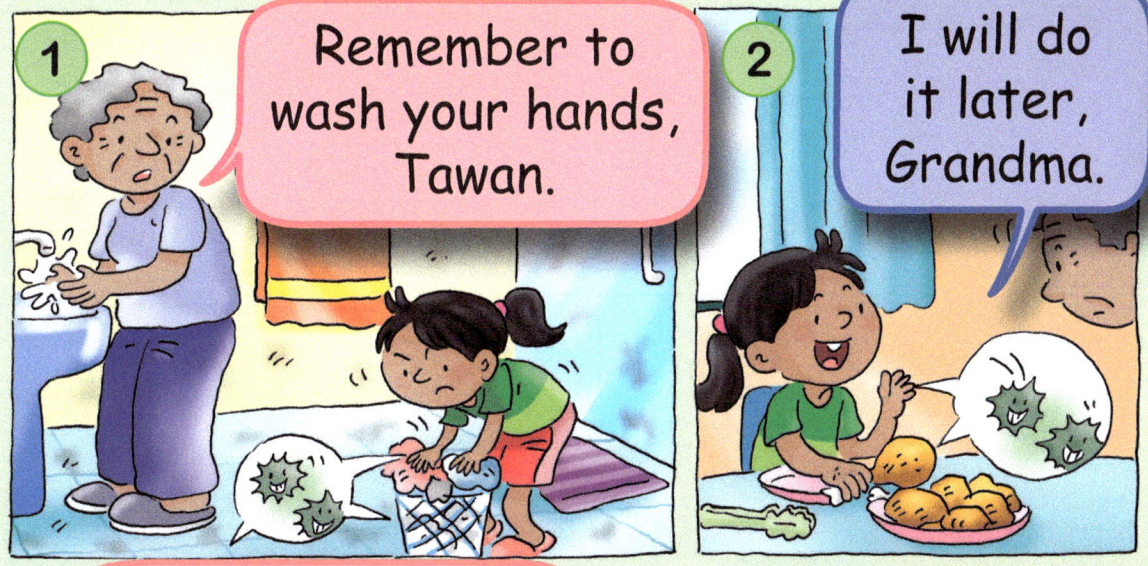

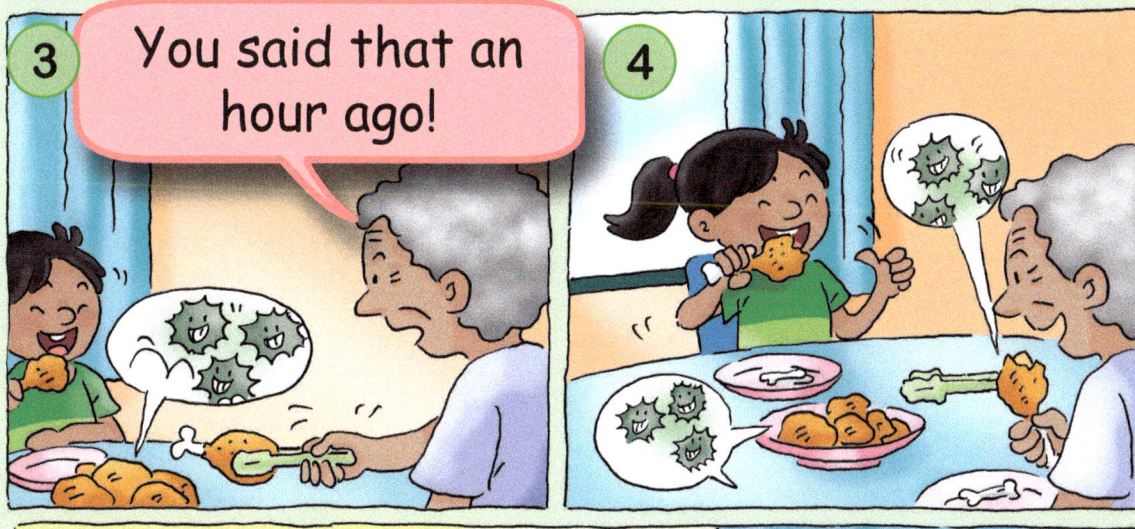

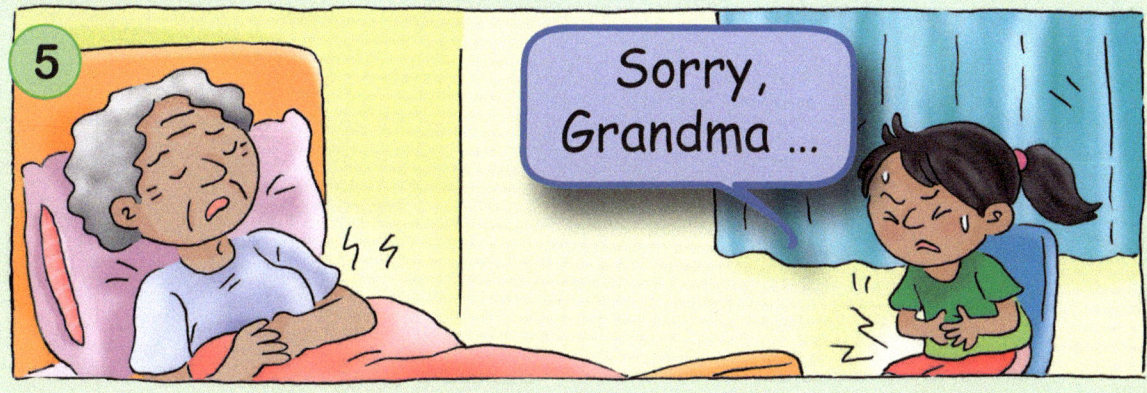

Learning Objectives: Pupils will be able to recognise that an unclean environment is a risk to healthy living for everyone. They will also learn how they can contribute to the prevention of the spread of diseases.

Germs are harmful because they spread diseases. Practise good hygiene to keep germs away.

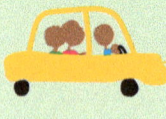 What made Tawan and her grandmother ill? Give three reasons in the space below. The pictures are clues.

Name: Class: Date:

Lesson 8

Germs Are Everywhere

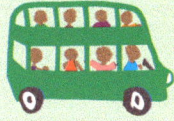 Look at the pictures below. Describe what you see.

1
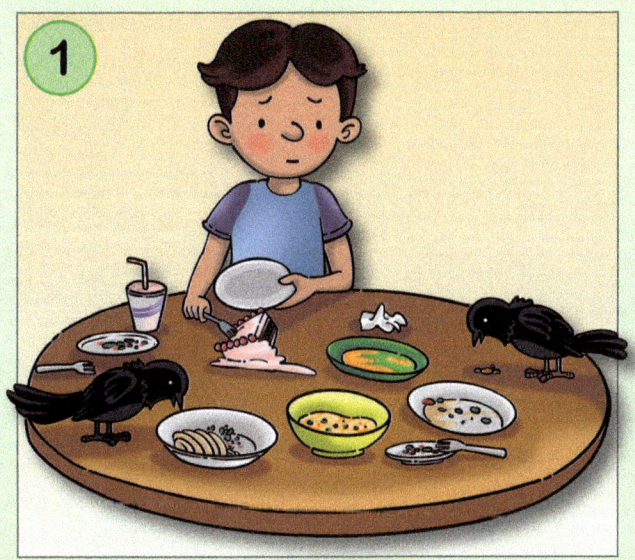

2
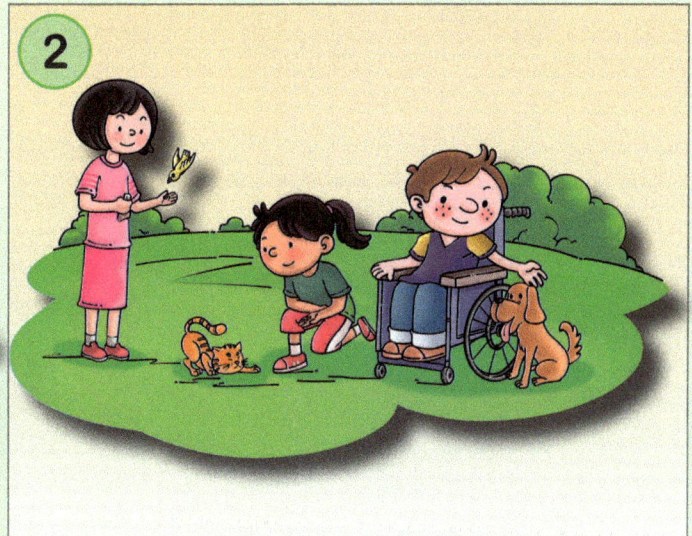

3
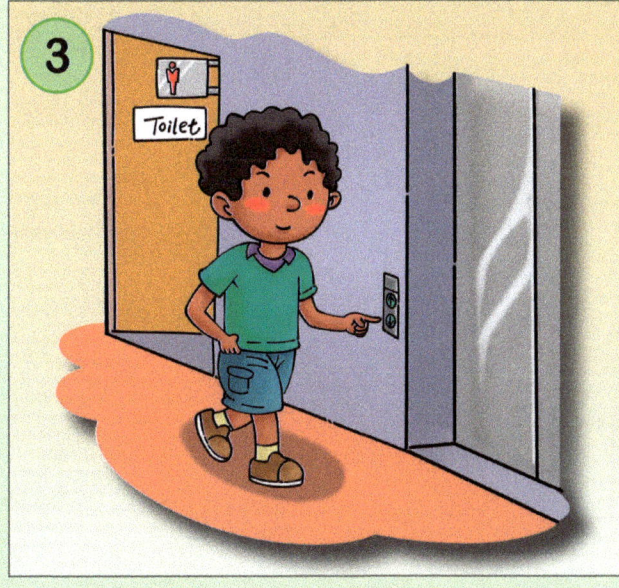

4
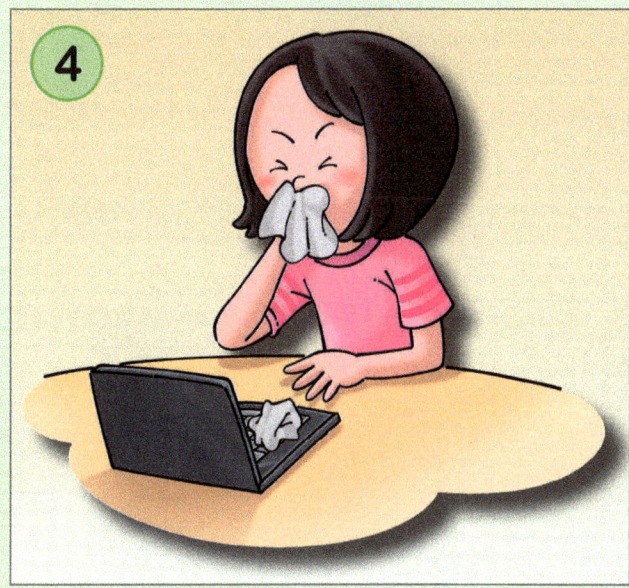

Learning Objectives: Pupils will be able to recognise that an unclean environment is a risk to healthy living for everyone. They will also learn how they can contribute to the prevention of the spread of diseases.

41

You have learnt that good hygiene keeps germs away. Another way to do that is to keep your surroundings clean.

Read what Haris, Eileen and Harold are saying.

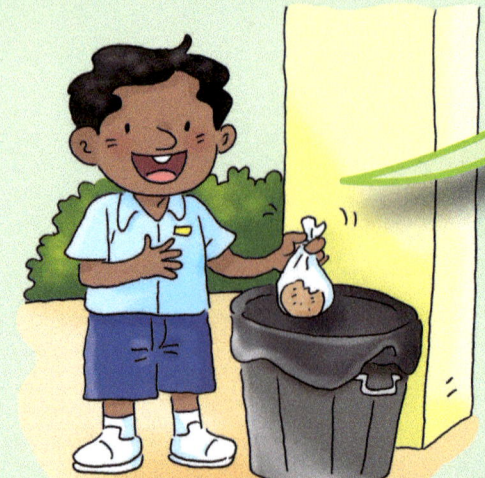

Throw unwanted food into a bin. If you can, put the food in a bag and tie it up.

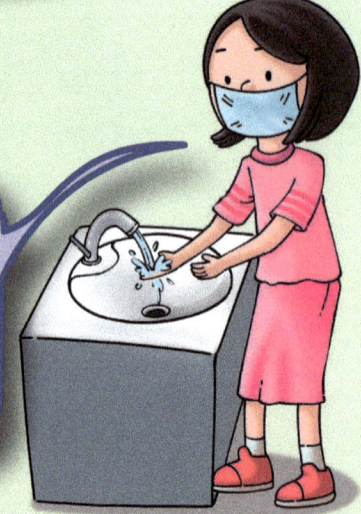

Put on a mask when you are having a cough or running nose. Wash your hands frequently, especially after using the toilet.

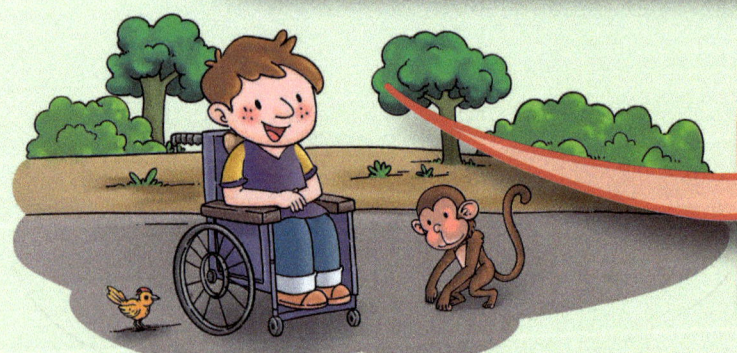

Do not feed cats, birds or monkeys. Food left behind can dirty the surroundings.

Can you remember learning about seven steps in hand hygiene? Practise the steps with your friends again!

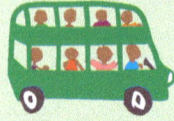

Lesson 9

Do Not Share Your Germs

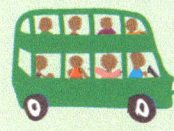 Follow the story in the comic strip below.

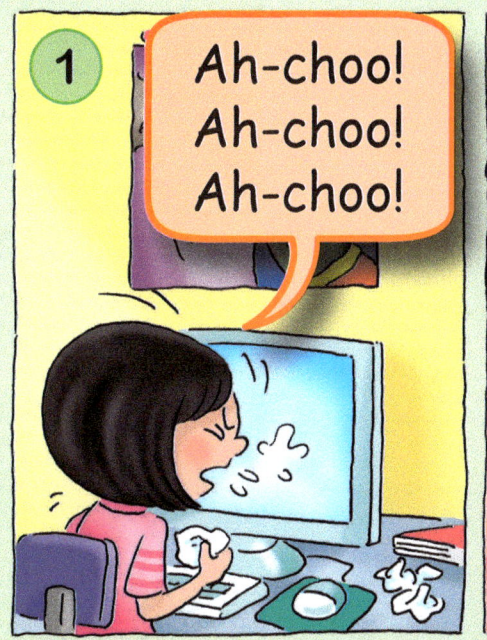

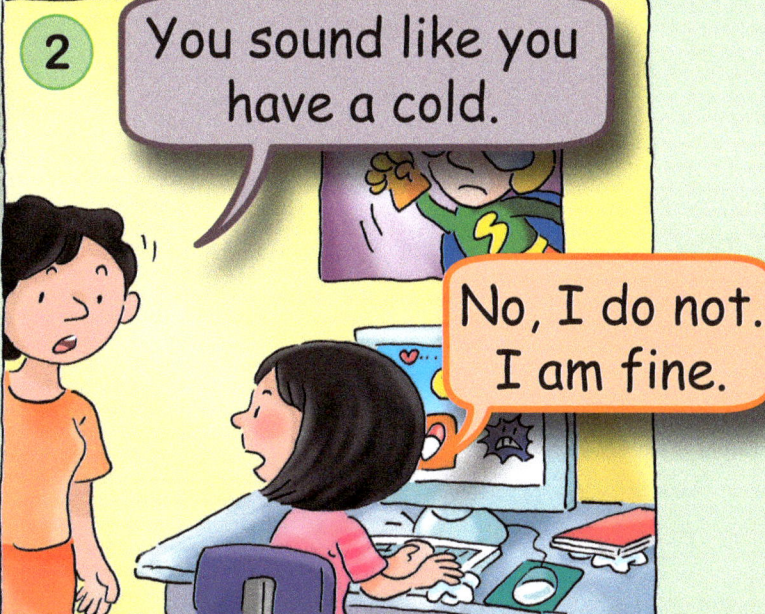

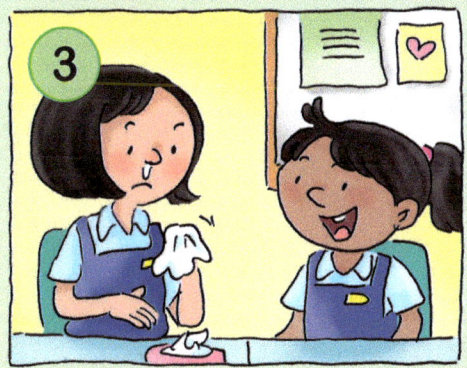

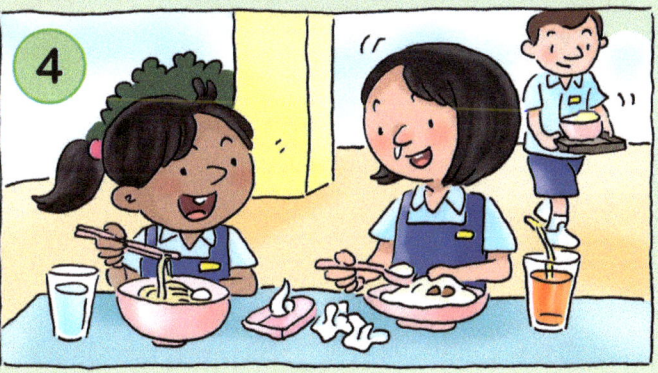

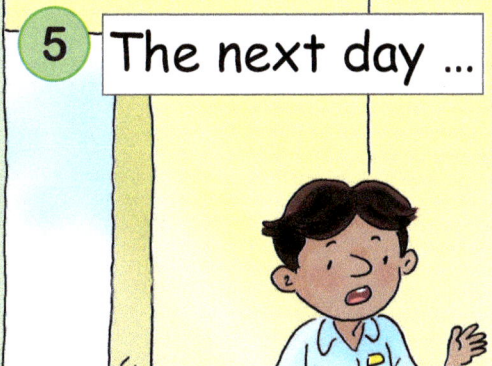

Learning Objectives: Pupils will be able to recognise that an unclean environment is a risk to healthy living for everyone. They will also learn how they can contribute to the prevention of the spread of diseases.

Have you ever gone to school when you were ill? How do you stop your germs from getting to others and making them ill?

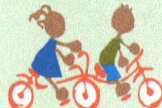 **Look at the pictures and complete.**

1. See a d_____ when you are ill.

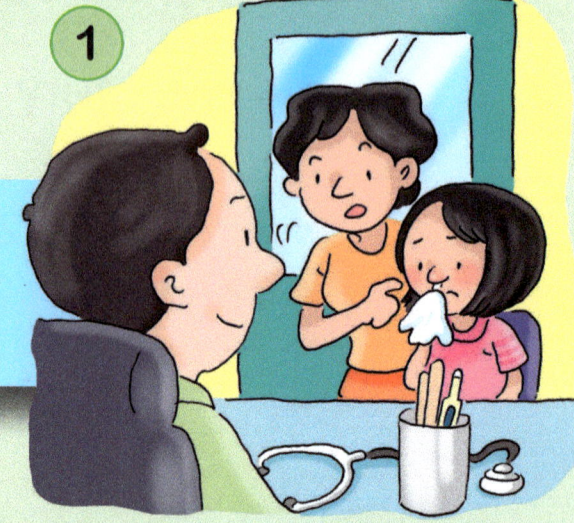

2. 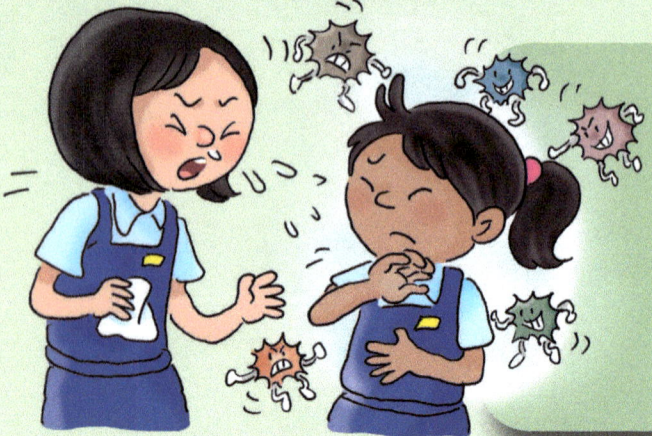 Rest at h____. Cover your mouth when you c_____ or s_____. Wear a mask.

3. Check your t_____ regularly. A fever is a symptom of the common flu, bird flu and dengue.

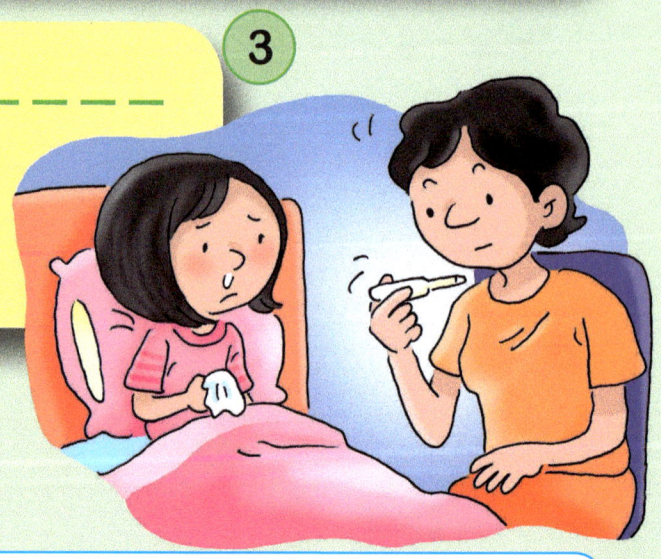

 **influenza or flu:** flu is an illness that affects breathing and it can be spread easily when an infected person coughs or sneezes.
avian flu or bird flu: avian flu is an influenza that mostly affects birds as it spreads from bird to bird. People who handle sick birds or birds who have died from avian flu have caught the flu from the animals.
dengue: this disease is spread by mosquitoes and the early signs are fever, rash and joint and muscle pain.

Emotional And Psychological Health

In this section, you will learn how to:

- manage your emotions;
- show care for others; and
- deal with bullying and teasing.

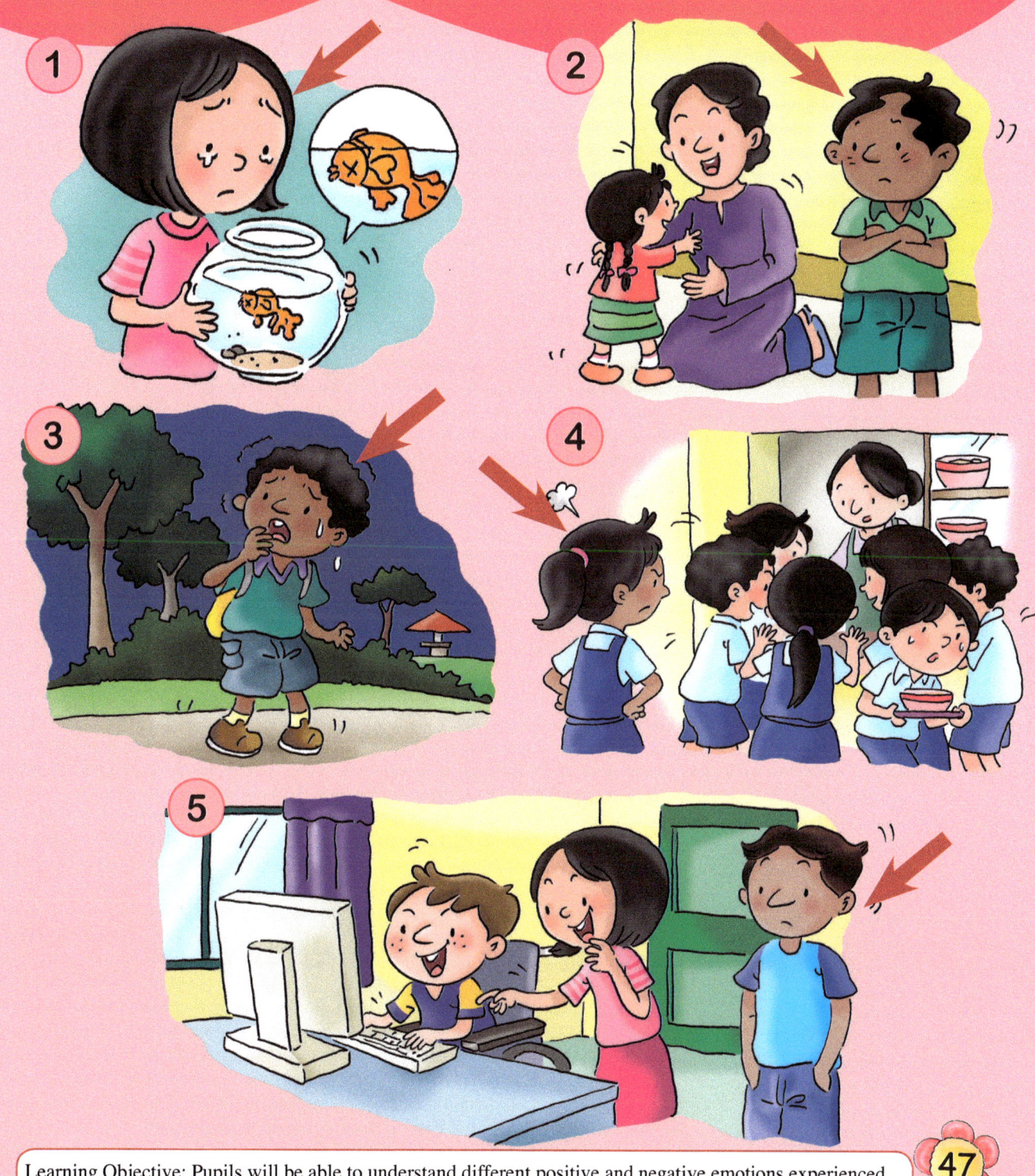

How would you feel if you were 1. Eileen, 2. Haris, 3. Ajit and 4. Lam? Match the feelings in the yellow bubbles with each picture.

1

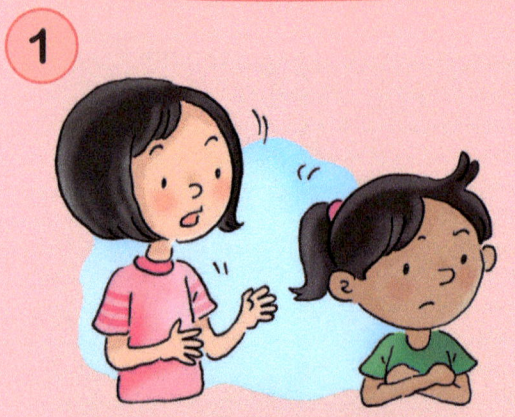

Your best friend ignored you.

2

Your classmates bullied you.

angry

sad

jealous

scared

insecure

3

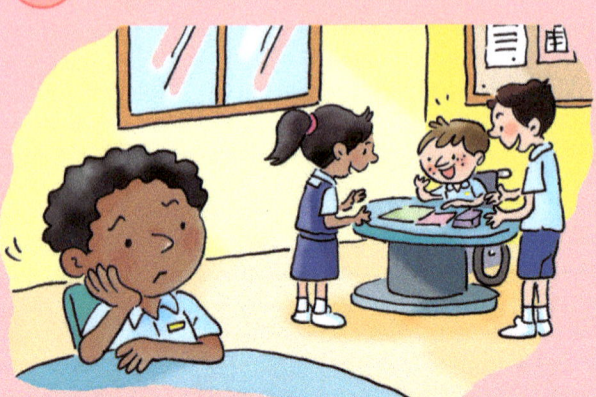

Your good friends left you out in an activity.

4

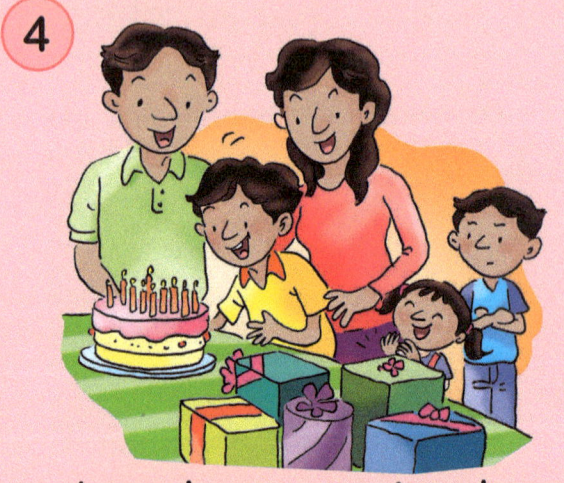

Your brother received many presents on his birthday.

It is all right to feel scared, angry, jealous and insecure. Grown-ups have these feelings too. However, it is important to know why we feel that way. We must understand what they can do to us if we are not careful.

Name: Class: Date: Lesson 2

Dealing With Anger

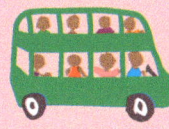 Read what the superfriends are saying.

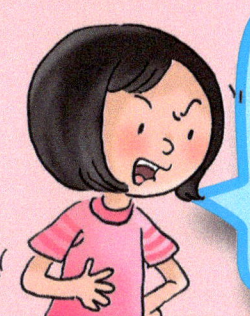 Ooh... I am so angry! I forgot to save my work on the computer again.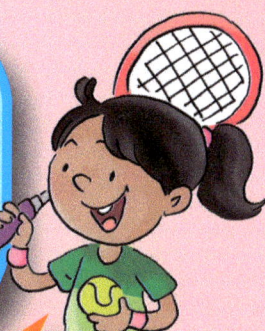

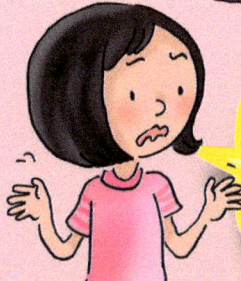 It is too hot for a swim.

Cheer up! When things go wrong, take a break. Go for a swim, a walk or a jog.

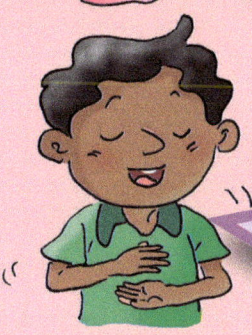 You could do some deep breathing to calm yourself down.

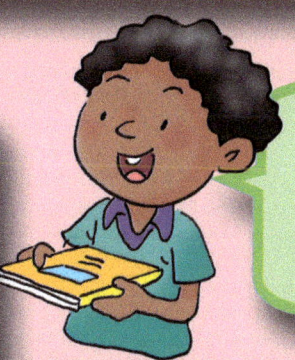 Or stay home and read a good book.

Music always makes me feel better!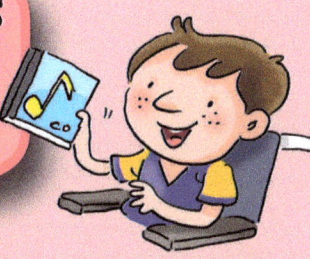

What do you do when things go wrong?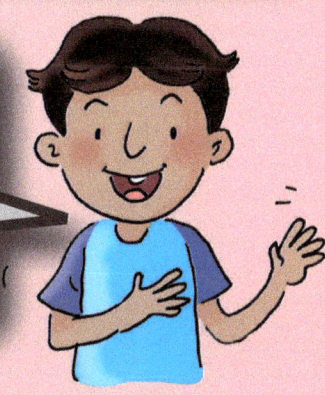

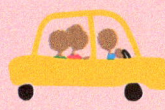 What can make you angry? Share about what you do when you feel angry.

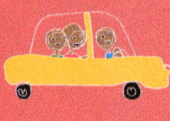 Eileen talked to her friends when she was angry. What would you do? Write or draw out your answers in the spaces below.

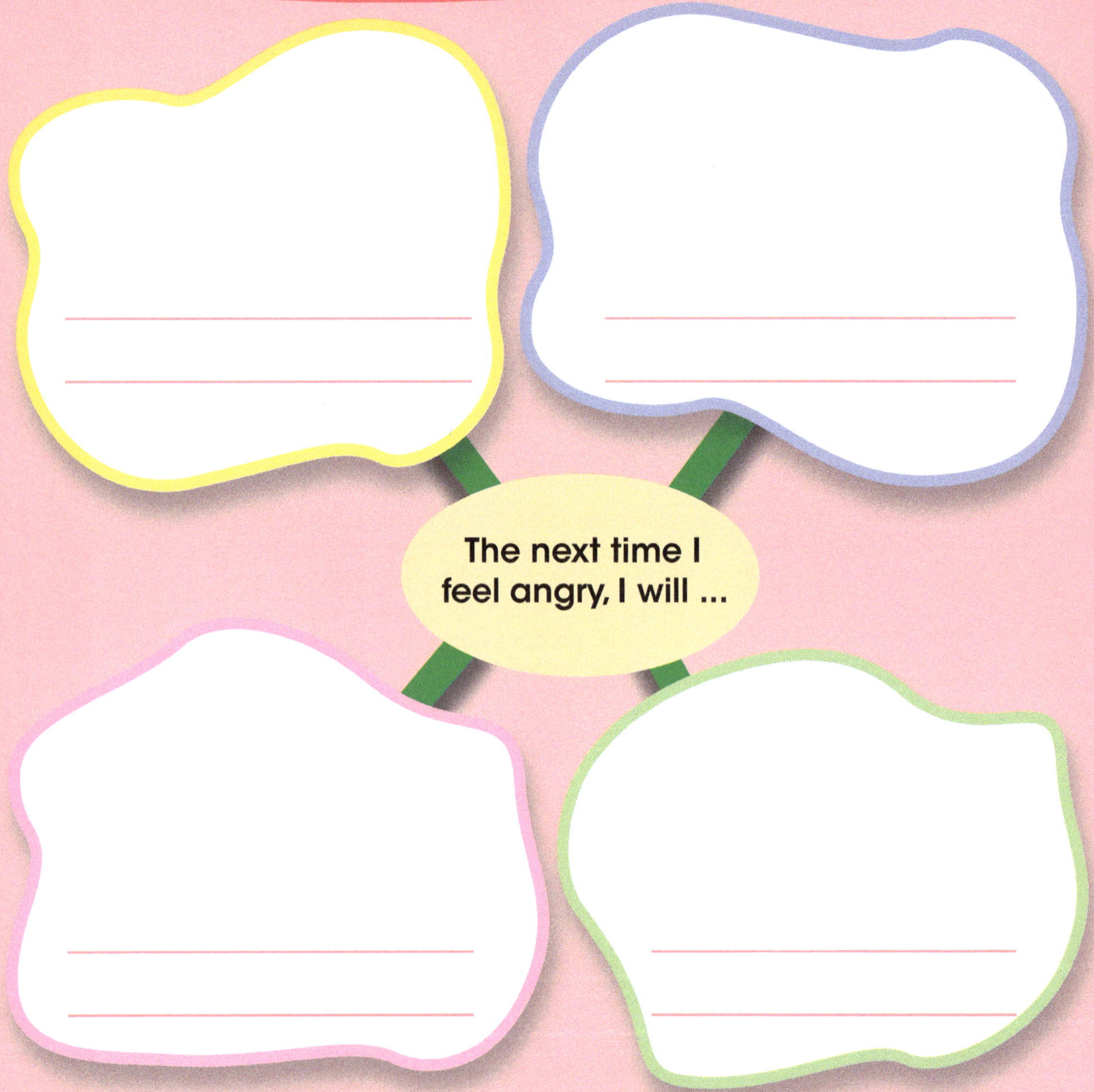

The next time I feel angry, I will ...

1. Pause and breathe deeply when you start to feel angry.
2. Do not try to solve the problem immediately. Wait for some time to pass.
3. Use this time to talk to your family, teachers or friends.
4. Think about the problem carefully and decide what to do about it.

Name: Class: Date: Lesson 3

Lam's Story

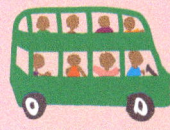 Follow the story in the comic strip below.

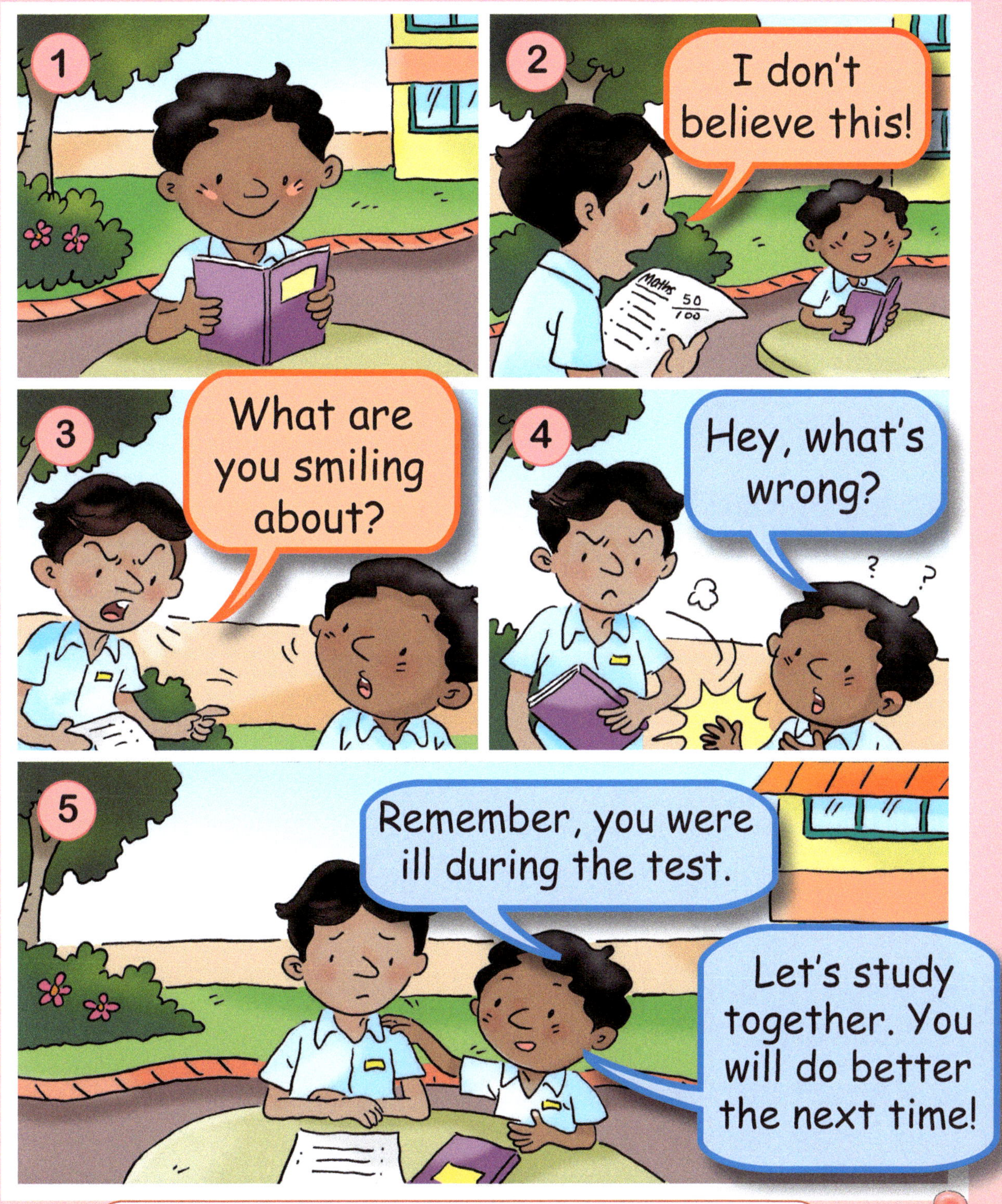

1

2 I don't believe this!

3 What are you smiling about?

4 Hey, what's wrong?

5 Remember, you were ill during the test. Let's study together. You will do better the next time!

Learning Objectives: Pupils will be able to understand how different emotions can affect others, and identify ways of managing negative emotions in positive ways.

When you feel bad about yourself, it helps to think about what you are good at.

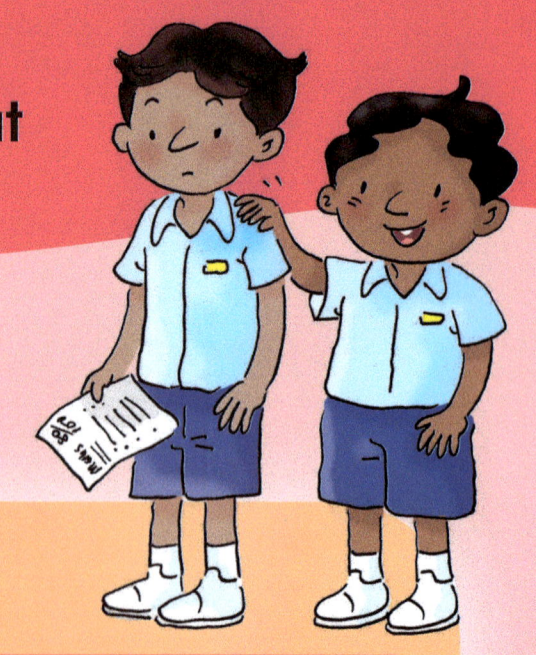

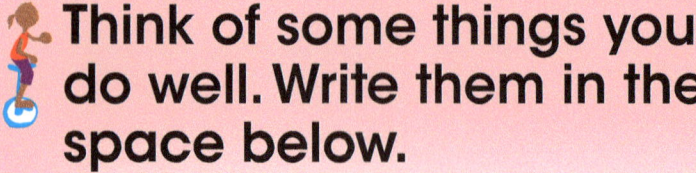 Think of some things you do well. Write them in the space below.

Whenever you feel you are not good enough, think about what you wrote above. You will feel better.

Read the words of encouragement below with your partner.

Words of Encouragement
- ✔ It is all right to try at something and not succeed the first few times.
- ✔ Understand why you did not succeed. Ask for help and try again.
- ✔ Remember: You did not fail, you just have not succeeded yet!

Name: Class: Date: Lesson 4

Caring For Others

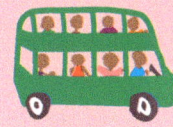 Look at the pictures below. Describe what Lam, Tawan and Ajit are doing.

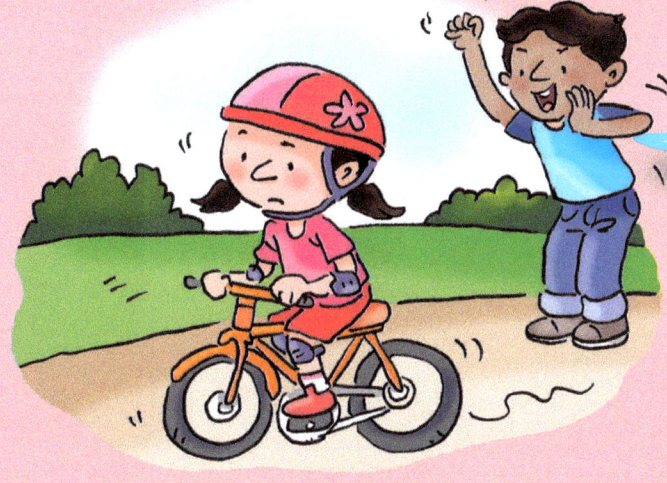

You can do it!

Let me help you, Grandma.

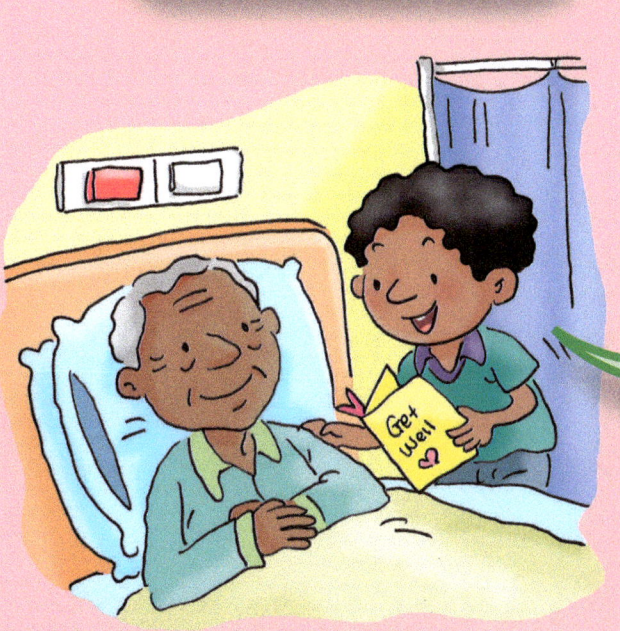

I will stay and keep you company, Grandpa.

Learning Objectives: Pupils will be able to explore different ways of developing healthy relationships with family members, peers and school leaders, and identify characteristics of positive and negative relationships.

You can show care for others through your actions, kind words and by spending time with them.

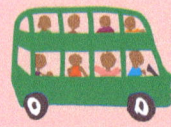 Think of a good deed you can do for your parent, teacher and friend. Write it in the space below.

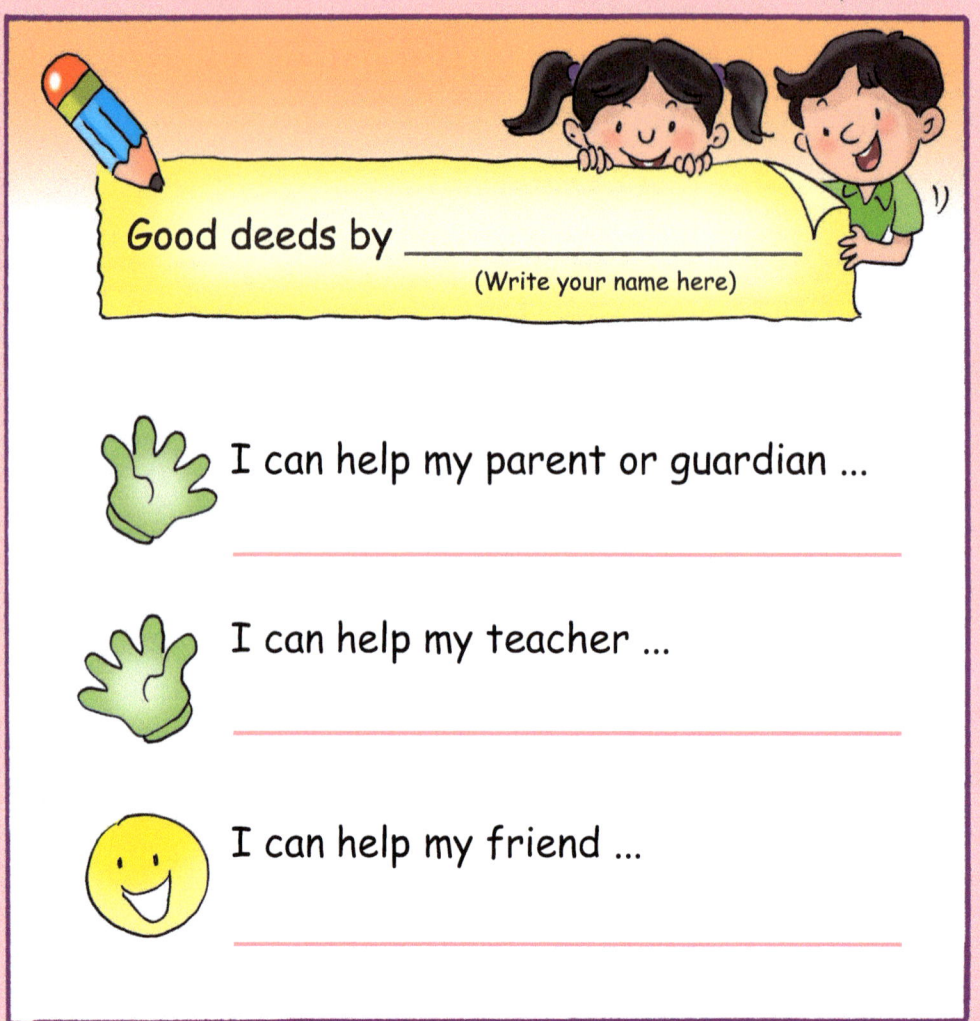

Good deeds by _____
(Write your name here)

I can help my parent or guardian ...
_____

I can help my teacher ...
_____

I can help my friend ...
_____

Be kind to others and be kind to yourself.
Be useful to others and be useful to yourself.

 Listen to different answers to these two questions:

- How can you be kind to others and to yourself?
- How can you be useful to others and to yourself?

Name: Class: Date:

Lesson 5

Crack The Code!

Help Haris find out the superfriends' secret to being such good friends. Listen carefully as your teacher reads. Circle '1' or '2'.

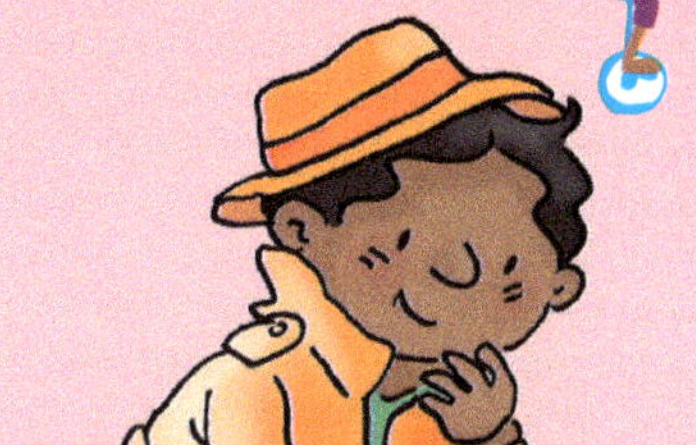

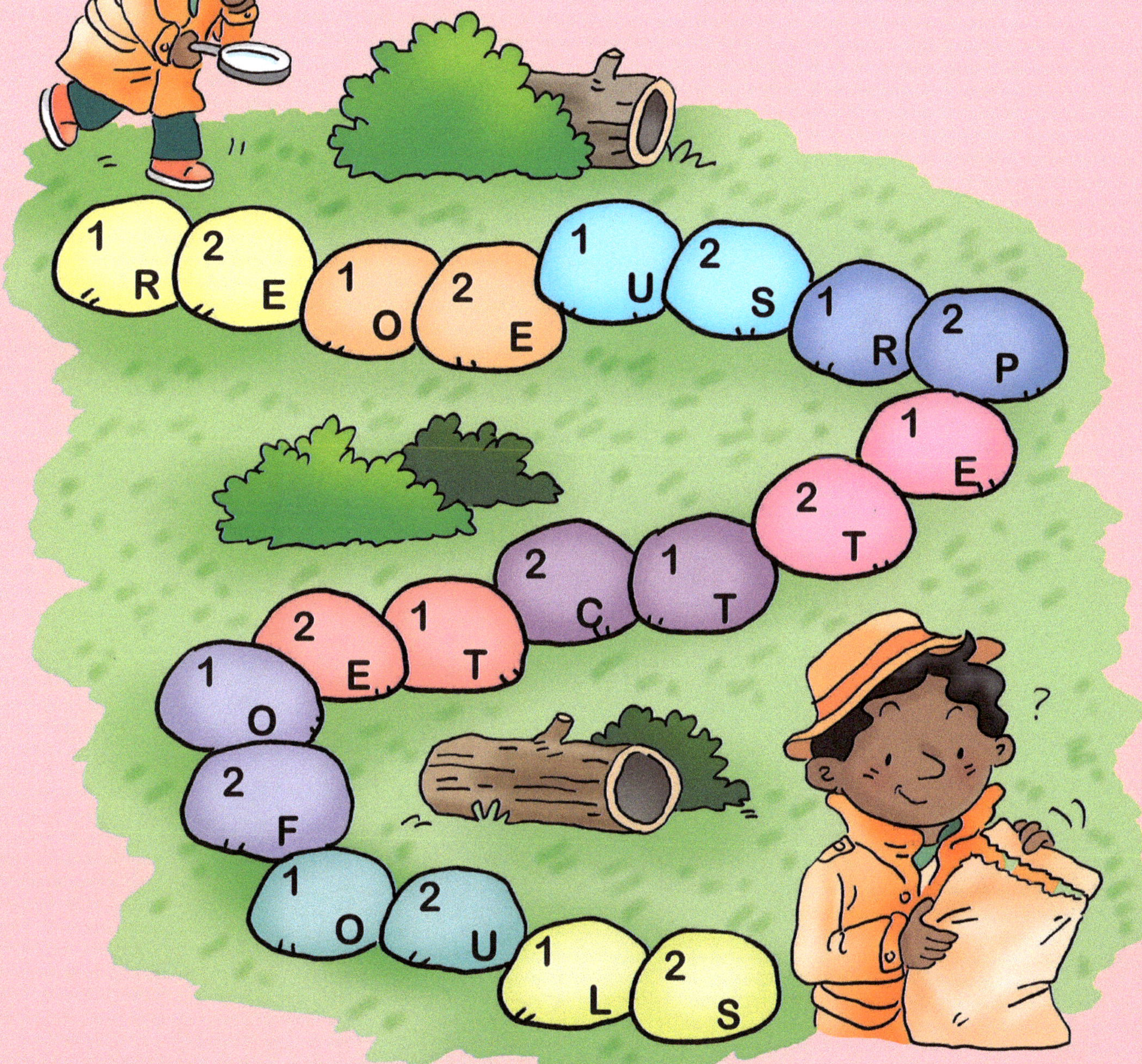

Learning Objective: Pupils will be able to explore different ways of developing healthy relationships with family members, peers and school leaders.

The secret to the superfriends can be found on the path on page 55.

In the correct order, write the letter beside each number you have circled.

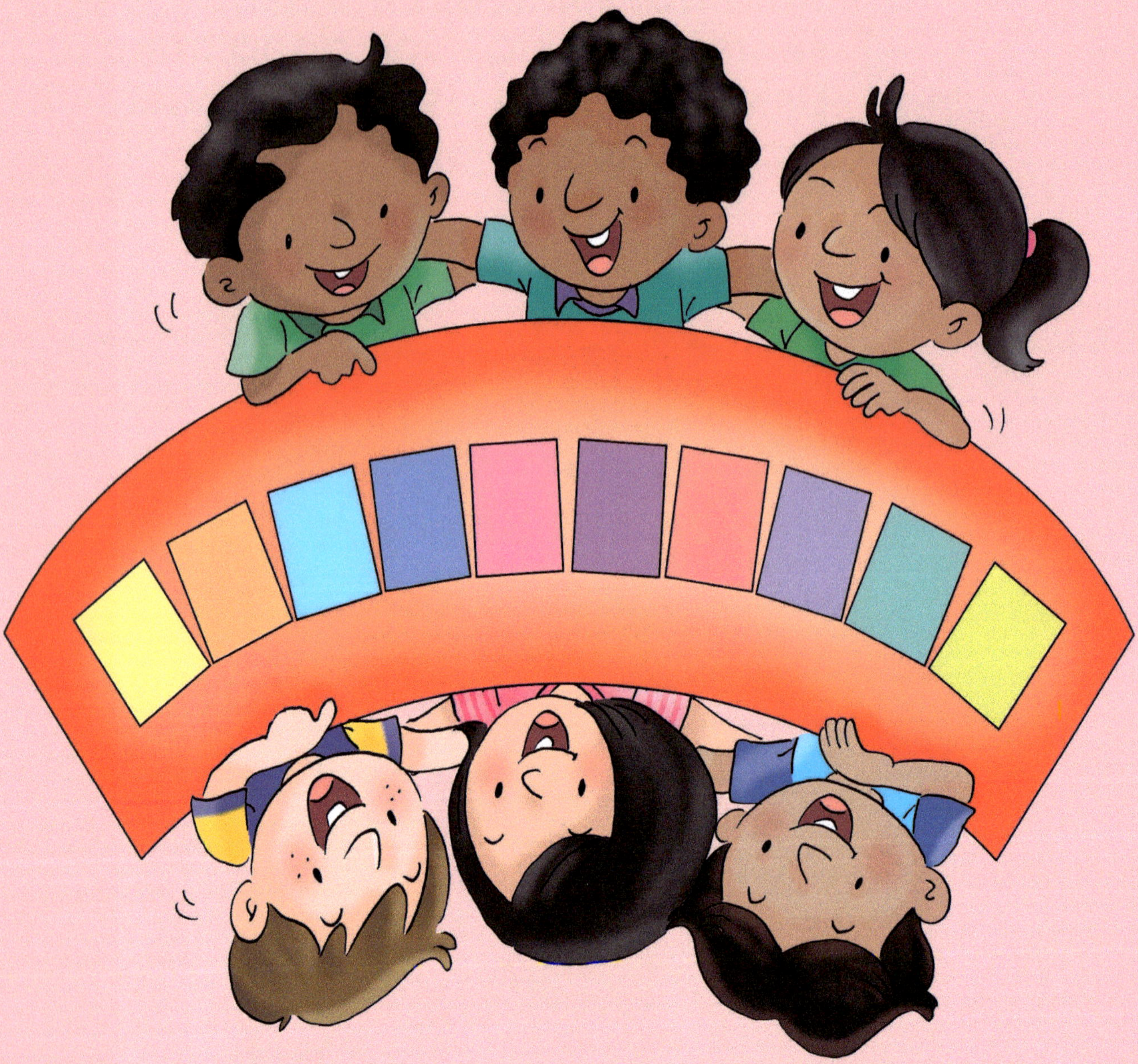

We are superfriends because we are
_____ of each other.

Name: Class: Date: Lesson 6

Wonderful Words

🚴 Trace the outline of your hand below. Cut it out. Write your name in the centre. Think of five things you can say to someone to show you care about him or her. Write them on the outline of each finger.

Learning Objective: Pupils will be able to explore different ways of developing healthy relationships with family members, peers and school leaders.

This page is left blank for the cutting exercise on the previous page.

Name: Class: Date:

Lesson 7

Leave Me Alone!

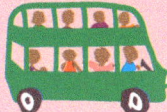 **Look at the pictures below. Describe what each of them shows.**

1
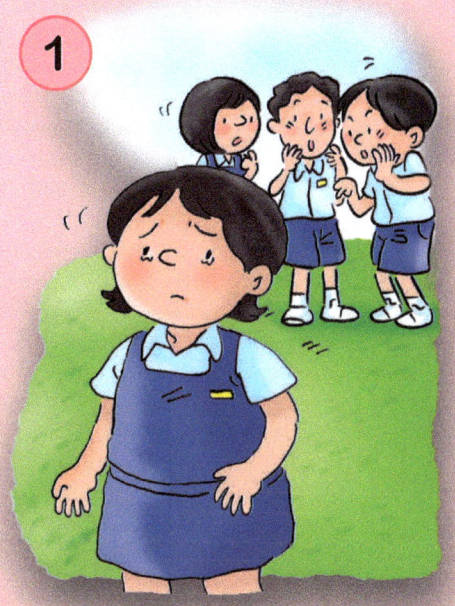

2
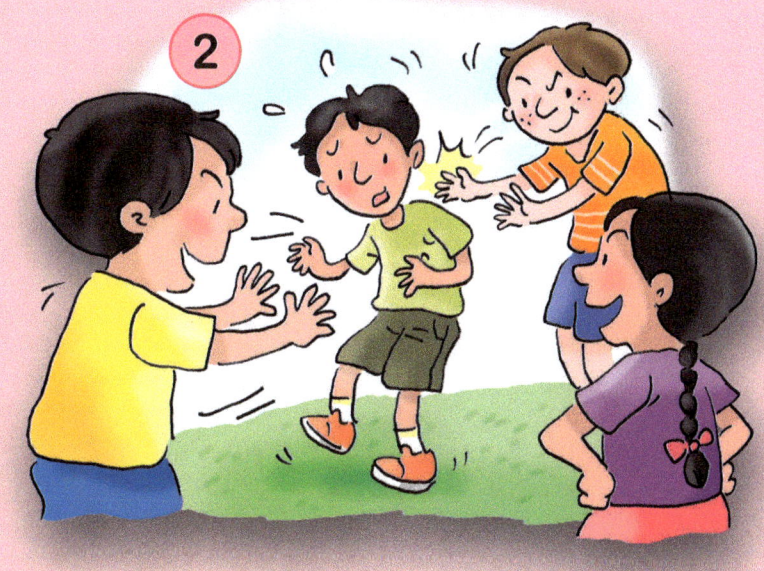

3
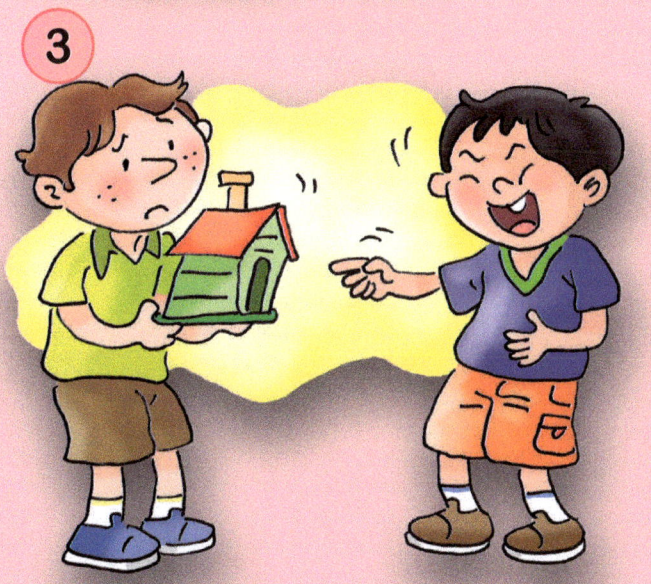

4
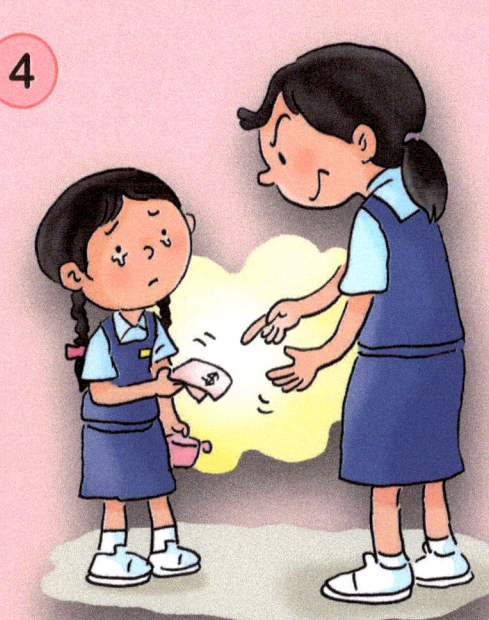

Learning Objective: Pupils will be able to identify characteristics of positive and negative relationships.

59

People who tease or bully others usually have their own problems. They say or do unkind things to make themselves feel important.

You should never argue with them or say unkind things in return.

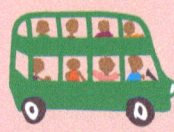 What should you do instead?

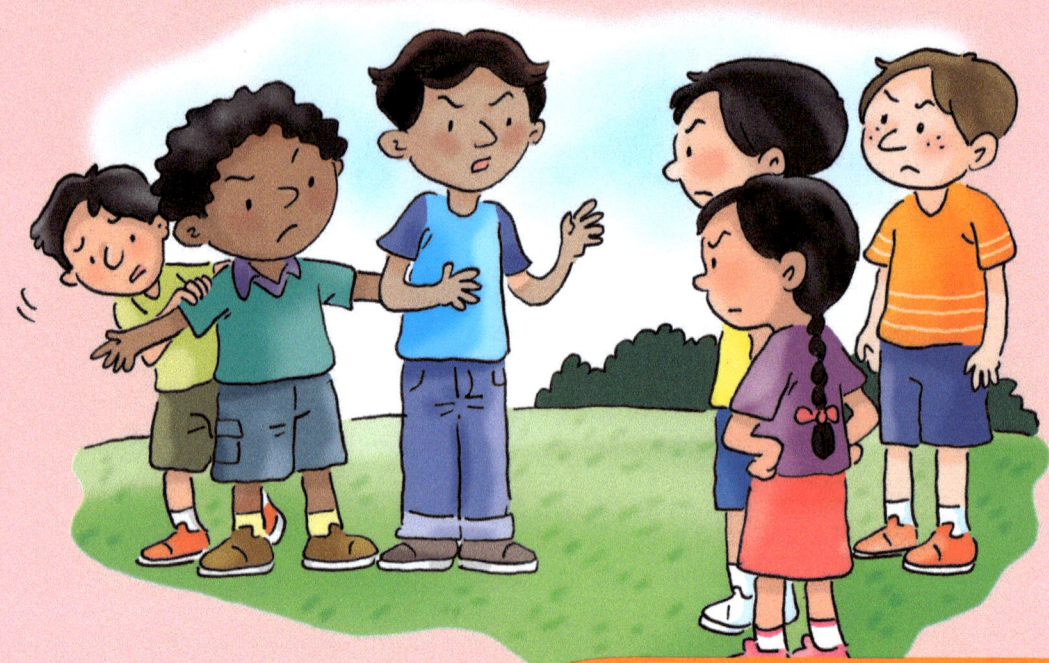

Pretend to agree with them?

Ask them to stop and say what they are doing is not funny?

Ignore them or walk away?

Talk to someone who can help?

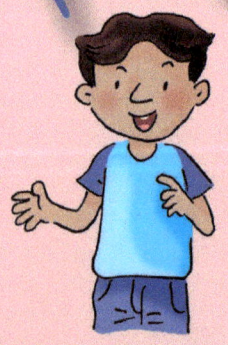 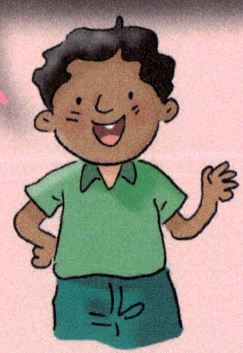 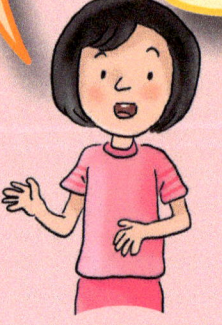 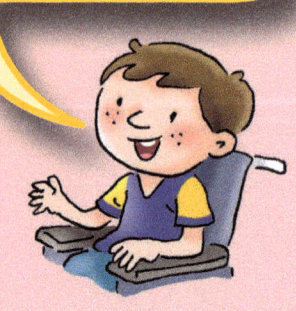

tease: to laugh at playfully or unkindly, or make jokes about a person.
bully: to use your strength to hurt or frighten people who are not as strong as you are.

Name: _____ Class: ___ Date: ___

Lesson 8

Bullying And Teasing

Have you done the following before? If you have, put a tick (✓) in one of the boxes. Show if you did it alone or with a group of people.

	Alone	In a Group
1. Tried to make someone feel bad.	☐	☐
2. Made fun of someone.	☐	☐
3. Called someone unkind names.	☐	☐
4. Threatened someone.	☐	☐
5. Done (1) to (4) on the Internet.	☐	☐

Learning Objective: Pupils will be able to identify characteristics of positive and negative relationships.

	Alone	In a Group
6. Hurt someone physically.	☐	☐
7. Made someone cry.	☐	☐
8. Said bad things about someone behind his or her back.	☐	☐
9. Tried to get others to do something unkind.	☐	☐
10. Laughed when others were bullied.	☐	☐

If you have put a tick (✓) in any of the boxes, you may have bullied or teased someone!

Stop! No one likes a person who bullies or teases unkindly. Think again before you do or say something hurtful to anyone.

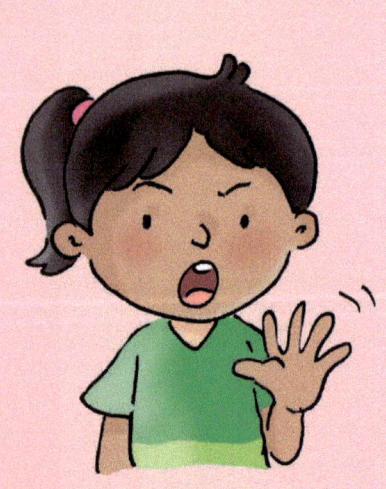
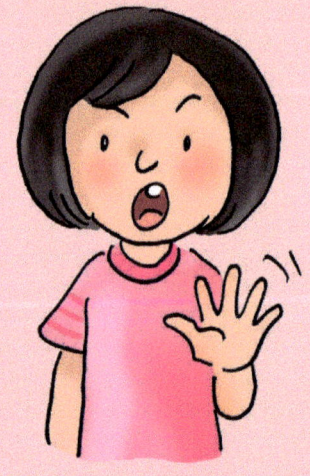
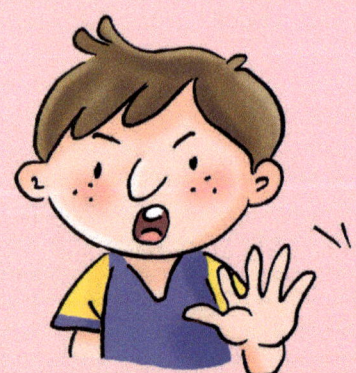

threaten: to tell someone you will harm him or her unless he or she does as you say.

How To Tackle Bullying

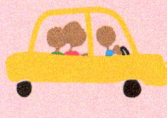 Take turns to read the following aloud. Think of two more points to add to the list.

1. Stand up and say loudly and firmly, 'Stop it! I do not like what you are doing to me.'
2. Walk away and move to a crowded area.
3. Tell your friend, teacher or parents about it.
4. Avoid being alone and avoid places where bullies hang out.
5. Stay calm, stand tall and be positive.

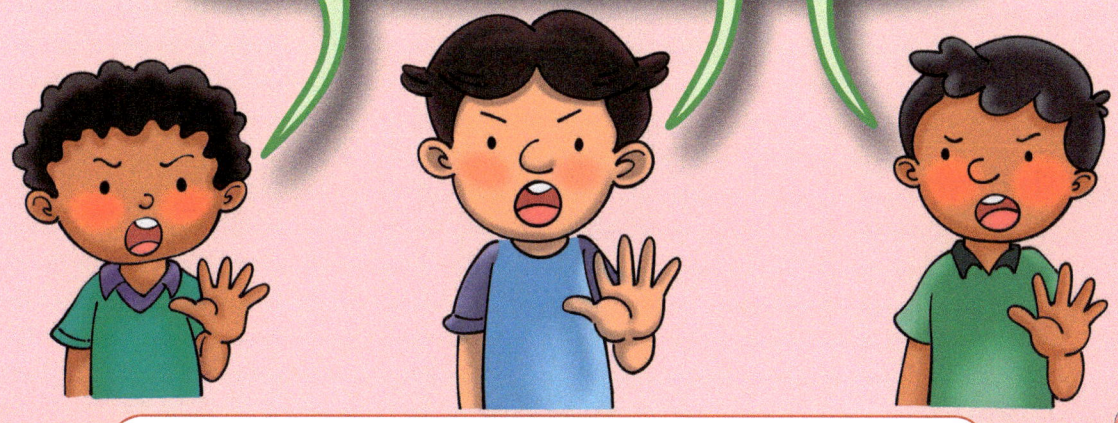

Say 'No!' to bullying!

Learning Objective: Pupils will be able to identify characteristics of positive and negative relationships.

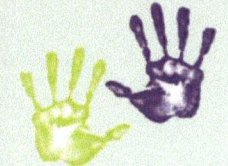 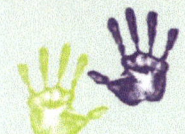

HANDS
are not for hitting

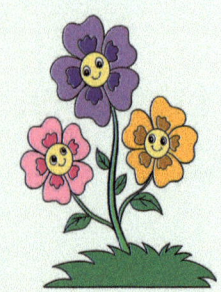 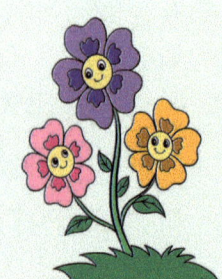

WORDS
are not for hurting

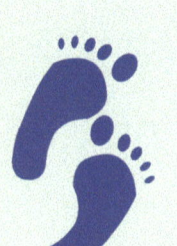 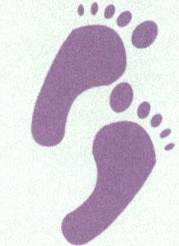

FEET
are not for kicking

Be kind instead!

With your partner, think of some ways you can use your hands, feet and words to help instead of hurt. Write them in the spaces below.

In school: _____

At home: _____

In public places: _____

NEW WORDS

Lesson: ____ Date: ____

MY LESSON TODAY ...
(Draw or write out the things you remember.)

Lesson: ____ Date: ____

MY LESSON TODAY ...
(Draw or write out the things you remember.)

Lesson: ____ Date: ____

MY LESSON TODAY ...
(Draw or write out the things you remember.)

Lesson: ____ Date: ____

MY LESSON TODAY ...
(Draw or write out the things you remember.)

Lesson: ____ Date: ____

MY LESSON TODAY ...
(Draw or write out the things you remember.)

MY LEARNING LOG

MY LEARNING LOG

NEW WORDS

Lesson: ____ Date: ____

MY LESSON TODAY …
(Draw or write out the things you remember.)

Lesson: ____ Date: ____

MY LESSON TODAY …
(Draw or write out the things you remember.)

Lesson: ____ Date: ____

MY LESSON TODAY …
(Draw or write out the things you remember.)

Lesson: ____ Date: ____

MY LESSON TODAY …
(Draw or write out the things you remember.)

Lesson: ____ Date: ____

MY LESSON TODAY …
(Draw or write out the things you remember.)

NEW WORDS

Lesson: Date:

MY LESSON TODAY ...
(Draw or write out the things you remember.)

Lesson: Date:

MY LESSON TODAY ...
(Draw or write out the things you remember.)

Lesson: Date:

MY LESSON TODAY ...
(Draw or write out the things you remember.)

Lesson: Date:

MY LESSON TODAY ...
(Draw or write out the things you remember.)

Lesson: Date:

MY LESSON TODAY ...
(Draw or write out the things you remember.)

MY LEARNING LOG

MY LEARNING LOG

NEW WORDS

Lesson: ___ Date: ___
MY LESSON TODAY …
(Draw or write out the things you remember.)

Lesson: ___ Date: ___
MY LESSON TODAY …
(Draw or write out the things you remember.)

Lesson: ___ Date: ___
MY LESSON TODAY …
(Draw or write out the things you remember.)

Lesson: ___ Date: ___
MY LESSON TODAY …
(Draw or write out the things you remember.)

Lesson: ___ Date: ___
MY LESSON TODAY …
(Draw or write out the things you remember.)

MY LEARNING LOG

NEW WORDS

Lesson: Date:

MY LESSON TODAY …
(Draw or write out the things you remember.)

Lesson: Date:

MY LESSON TODAY …
(Draw or write out the things you remember.)

Lesson: Date:

MY LESSON TODAY …
(Draw or write out the things you remember.)

Lesson: Date:

MY LESSON TODAY …
(Draw or write out the things you remember.)

Lesson: Date:

MY LESSON TODAY …
(Draw or write out the things you remember.)

MY LEARNING LOG

NEW WORDS

Lesson: Date:

MY LESSON TODAY ...
(Draw or write out the things you remember.)

Lesson: Date:

MY LESSON TODAY ...
(Draw or write out the things you remember.)

Lesson: Date:

MY LESSON TODAY ...
(Draw or write out the things you remember.)

Lesson: Date:

MY LESSON TODAY ...
(Draw or write out the things you remember.)

Lesson: Date:

MY LESSON TODAY ...
(Draw or write out the things you remember.)